Sonography of the Infant's Hip

Reinhard Graf · Claudia Maizen
Tamara Seidl

Sonography of the Infant's Hip

Principles, implementation and therapeutic consequences

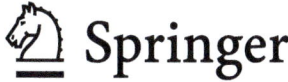 Springer

Reinhard Graf
Pediatric Orthopedics
LKH Stolzalpe
Murau, Austria

Claudia Maizen
Trauma and Orthopaedics
Royal London Hospital
London, UK

Tamara Seidl
Pediatric Orthopedics
Klinikum Herford
Herford, Nordrhein-Westfalen, Germany

ISBN 978-3-031-71948-6   ISBN 978-3-031-71949-3   (eBook)
https://doi.org/10.1007/978-3-031-71949-3

Translation from the German language edition: "Sonographie der Säuglingshüfte 7. Auflage" by Reinhard Graf et al., © 2022 Georg Thieme Verlag KG 2022. Published by Thieme. All Rights Reserved.

This Springer imprint is published by the registered company Springer Nature Switzerland AG
The registered company address is: Gewerbestrasse 11, 6330 Cham, Switzerland

If disposing of this product, please recycle the paper.

Introduction

When hip ultrasound was first presented at a conference after years of research in 1980, it was met with laughter: "Graf with his acetabular roof!" It was not foreseeable at the time that hip sonography would be used worldwide today. However, this was only possible through continuous development and analysis of every mistake that was made over the years. It is all the more surprising that modified techniques are now leading to mistakes that were made 30 years ago, resulting in the statement: "Hip sonography is not safe, and it is not reproducible."

This book is a translation of the seventh edition of the German book on Hip Ultrasound of the infant hip. The content of the book has been tidied up with each edition over the years and lengthy explanations were omitted in favour of facts that are now accepted by the scientific community. For those interested in the science of DDH hip ultrasound, this edition of the book together with the references to the literature fully cover the topic. Important points are repeated multiple times from various perspectives.

With today's standards, hip sonography is not only suitable for early diagnosis of dislocated hips, but also a preventive tool for the development of dislocation through early diagnosis and early treatment. As a result, the recommendations for ultrasound-guided treatment and newborn screening have been modified, and the imaging technique has been continuously improved. Currently, computer-assisted examination techniques are also developed.

At first glance, the course syllabus may seem basic, but it has been developed over decades through experience with courses in many different countries and is intended to be a guide for standardized training.

This is the first English edition of the textbook on Graf Hip Ultrasound and should be a helpful resource for beginners, learning the method for the first time, as well as a reference for advanced practitioners all over the world (www.learninghospital.com).

We would like to thank Dr. Sally Scott for proofreading this first English edition of the book.

> "After holding firmly to a certain way of doing things, one should pause and examine if their mind has become stagnant." - Henry Ford

An online version of the DDH Hip Ultrasound course in German and English by Prof. Graf in collaboration with Dr. Maizen are available on: www.learninghospital.com

Stolzalpe, Austria   Reinhard Graf
London, UK   Claudia Maizen
Bielefeld, Germany   Tamara Seidl

March 2024

Contents

1 From Congenital Dislocation of the Hip to Developmental
    Dislocation of the Hip 1
    1.1 History 1
    1.2 Incidence 1
    1.3 Timing of Treatment 1
    1.4 Overview of Diagnostic Tests 1
        1.4.1 Clinical Examination 1
        1.4.2 Radiological Diagnosis 2
        1.4.3 Magnetic Resonance Imaging (MRI). 2
        1.4.4 Ultrasonography. 3
    1.5 The Current State of Hip Sonography Worldwide. 4
        1.5.1 Current Problems 5
        1.5.2 Examination Techniques 5
        1.5.3 Screening 6
    References. 7

2 Hip Ultrasound Technique, Equipment, and Image
    Projection. 9
    2.1 Equipment 9
        2.1.1 Transducer 9
        2.1.2 Device Settings and Frequencies 10
        2.1.3 Hip Sonography-Specific Equipment 10
    2.2 Documentation. 11
        2.2.1 Standard Image Criteria. 11
        2.2.2 Methodological Image Criteria 11
    References. 13

3 The Pillars of Hip Sonography 15
    3.1 Development of the Hip Joint 15
    3.2 Direction of the Ultrasound Beam and the Soft Tissue
        Overlying the Hip 16
    3.3 Femoral Neck and Femoral Head 17
        3.3.1 Anatomy and Development 17
        3.3.2 Proximal Part of the Femur 18
        3.3.3 Femoral Head and Ossific Nucleus 19
        3.3.4 Structures Surrounding the Femoral Head. 24
        3.3.5 Summary 26

3.4 Acetabular Fossa and Acetabular Roof 26
    3.4.1 Acetabular Fossa 26
    3.4.2 Cartilaginous Acetabular Roof. 28
    3.4.3 Boundaries and Special Sonographic
          Structure of the Hyaline Cartilage Roof 28
    3.4.4 Summary 31
3.5 Pathology of the Acetabulum. 31
    3.5.1 Morphological Changes During the Dislocation
          Process. 32
    3.5.2 Histological Changes at the Acetabulum 32
References. 35

4 Step-by-Step Approach to Hip Sonography 37
4.1 Anatomical Identification (Checklist I) 37
    4.1.1 Chondro-Osseous Border, Femoral Head,
          Synovial Fold, and Joint Capsule. 37
    4.1.2 The Labrum 37
    4.1.3 Standard Sequence. 38
    4.1.4 Turning Point 39
    4.1.5 Checklist I 40
4.2 Usability Check 40
    4.2.1 The Standard Plane 40
    4.2.2 Usability Check 43
    4.2.3 Checklist II. 44
    4.2.4 Exceptions from the Standard Plane 44
    4.2.5 Echoes Within the Acetabular Fossa 45
4.3 Summary 46
References. 47

5 Positioning, Scanning Technique, and Possible Errors 49
5.1 Advantages of the Recommended Examination
    Technique. 50
5.2 Positioning the Baby 50
5.3 Clinic Set-up in Practice 50
    5.3.1 Equipment 50
    5.3.2 Position of the Examiner and the
          Accompanying Adult. 50
    5.3.3 Instructions and Guidance to the
          Accompanying Adult. 51
5.4 Scanning Technique. 53
    5.4.1 Right Hip Joint. 53
    5.4.2 Left Hip Joint. 55
5.5 Summary 56
5.6 Possible Sources of Error. 56
    5.6.1 Problems Related to the Organization and to
          the Position 56
    5.6.2 Tilting Errors 57

6   Measurement Techniques and Possible Sources of Errors   61
   6.1   Angle Measurement.   61
   6.2   Bony Roof Line   61
      6.2.1   Definition   61
      6.2.2   Measurement Errors.   62
   6.3   Baseline   64
      6.3.1   Definition   64
      6.3.2   Problems   64
   6.4   Cartilage Roof Line   65
      6.4.1   Definition   65
      6.4.2   Measurement Errors.   65
   6.5   Bony Roof Angle α and Cartilage Roof Angle β   66
   6.6   Summary   67
   References.   68

7   Classification by Type of Sonograms of the Hip Joint.   69
   7.1   Basic Principles   69
   7.2   Sonometer and Maturation Curve   70
   7.3   Sonographic Hip Types and Differentiation   71
      7.3.1   Hip Types.   71
      7.3.2   Differentiation Between Structural
             Pathological Changes and Ossification   80
   7.4   Summary and Conclusion   82
   References.   83

8   Evaluation of Hip Sonograms   85
   8.1   Documentation of Name, Date of Birth, Affected Joint,
       and Patient's Age   85
   8.2   Checklist I   85
   8.3   Checklist II.   85
   8.4   Description and Reporting.   85
   8.5   Measurement Technique   87
   8.6   Determination of the Final Type   87
   8.7   Therapeutic Consequences.   87

9   Dynamic Stress Test   89
   9.1   Clinical Instability and Sonographic Instability   89
   9.2   Conducting the Stress Test.   89
   9.3   Elastic Whipping   91
   9.4   Typing of Sonographically Unstable Hip Joints   92
   9.5   Typing of Unstable Hip Joints   92

10   Special Features and Sources of Errors   95
   10.1   Questions of Nomenclature   95
   10.2   Most Common Errors in Practice   96
      10.2.1   Errors during the Examination   96
      10.2.2   Errors during the Anatomical Identification
             and the Usability Check   96

10.3   Neglecting the Patient's Age   98
       10.3.1   Age Limit for Hip Ultrasound.   98
       10.3.2   Premature Infants   98
Reference   98

11   Ultrasound-Based Treatment   99
11.1   Maturation Curve   99
11.2   Basic Treatment Principles Based on Biomechanical
       Aspects   99
11.3   Treatment Goals   99
11.4   Stages of Treatment 100
       11.4.1   Preparation 100
       11.4.2   Reduction 100
       11.4.3   Retention 102
       11.4.4   Maturation Phase 103
11.5   Deviation from the Treatment Algorithm in Newborns 107
11.6   Treatment Failures 109
       11.6.1   Late Diagnosis with Subsequent Delayed
                Start of Treatment 109
       11.6.2   Inappropriate Choice of Treatment for the Stage . . . 109
       11.6.3   Lack of Parental Compliance 109
11.7   Follow-up Intervals 109
11.8   Summary 110
References 110

12   Course Programme and Syllabus 111
12.1   Fundamentals of Hip Sonography 111
12.2   Anatomical Identification 112
12.3   Usability Check 113
12.4   Hip Types 114
12.5   Reporting 115
12.6   Description 116
12.7   Measurement Technique 117
12.8   Sonometer 118
12.9   Instability and Elastic Whipping 119
12.10 Tilting Errors 120
12.11 Scanning Technique 120

13   Practical Exercises 123
13.1   Part 1: Questions 123
       13.1.1   Identification of Anatomical Structures 123
       13.1.2   Usability Check (Lower Limb, Plane, Labrum) 123
13.2   Part 2: Answers 127
       13.2.1   Identification of Anatomical Structures 127
       13.2.2   Usability Check (Lower Limb, Plane, Labrum) 127

From Congenital Dislocation of the Hip to Developmental Dislocation of the Hip

1.1 History

The history of the diagnosis and treatment of congenital hip dislocation reads like a detective story. In Greek mythology, Homer described a number of deformed creatures, such as Hephaistos, who was ridiculed for his limp by the gods. Hippocrates knew about congenital dislocation of the hip and described different variations of dislocation and the symptom of waddling gait. As traumatic hip dislocation was already widely known, congenital hip dislocation was considered a distinct entity, and it was thought to be dislocation in utero. It was believed that the atrophy of muscles and bones was caused by the lack of pressure and counter-pressure within the dislocated joint. Interestingly, Hippocrates in his work distanced himself from the general attitude at the time, advocating for the early treatment of babies with hip dislocation. Around 100 years BC extension for the treatment of congenital hip dislocation was already known and practised. For centuries, doctors have dealt with the problem of congenital hip dislocation in different ways, leading to confusion and misunderstanding. For example, doctors in ancient Persia and Arabia traditionally treated congenital hip dislocation, which was thought to be caused by an effusion in the hip joint, with a branding iron.

1.2 Incidence

Congenital dislocation of the hip is the commonest congenital deformity of the musculoskeletal system. In central Europe, 1 to 5% of newborns are affected.

1.3 Timing of Treatment

The ultimate goal is early diagnosis in order to achieve complete reversal of the patho-anatomical deformity with early treatment. According to the studies of Ortolani [1], Rosen [2], and Barlow [3], early detection of disorders of hip maturation immediately after birth can consistently enable almost complete resolution of the anatomical changes if appropriate treatment is initiated promptly. However, according to Becker [4] and Schultheiss [5], starting treatment after the first 3 months of life only results in complete resolution in about two-thirds of cases.

1.4 Overview of Diagnostic Tests

1.4.1 Clinical Examination

The need for clinical examination remains undisputed, although its value has fundamentally changed in the era of hip sonography. Even before the introduction of hip sonography, the reliability of clinical diagnosis, which depends on many subjective factors, was doubted [6–8]. The undetectable so-called silent cases of hip dysplasia significantly hinder timely diagnosis [9–11]. Clinical signs such as movement restrictions, asymmetry of the skin folds, Roser-Ortolani sign [12], Barlow sign [3], and Dry-Click phenomenon are not sensitive enough reliably to identify hip dislocation or dysplasia.

Learning point
Using the clinical examination alone is insufficient for the reliable detection of disorders of hip maturation.

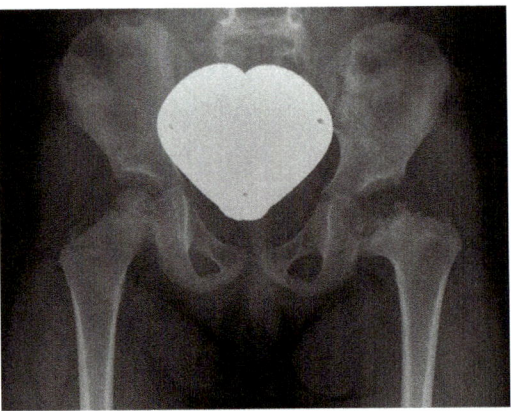

Fig. 1.1 Development of avascular necrosis of the left hip following closed reduction of a left-sided hip dislocation first diagnosed at just under 6 months of age

1.4.2 Radiological Diagnosis

The interpretation of hip X-rays in the neonatal period is difficult due to the limited information obtained from an image that only shows the ossified parts of the hip joint [13], it is not without controversy [14–16]. As a result, an X-ray examination is generally only indicated after the third to fourth month of life. Later X-rays should be performed for previously treated hip joints to rule out avascular necrosis of the femoral head or late dysplasia, for example, at the age of 2 years, before starting school, prepuberty, and after the completion of growth (Fig. 1.1). Arthrography, which can show the non-ossified parts and soft tissues of the hip joint, is comparable in diagnostic ability to hip sonography (Fig. 1.2). However, hip arthrography has mainly been replaced by hip sonography. Nonetheless, hip arthrography has significantly contributed to the understanding of the pathomechanics of the dislocation process [10, 17–21].

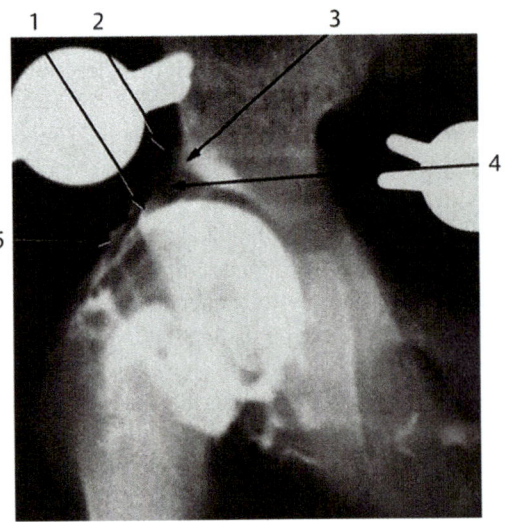

Fig. 1.2 Arthrography of the right hip. (Cadaver specimen, 1 = labrum, 2 = proximal, perichondrium, 3 = bony rim, 4 = hyaline cartilage roof, 5 = joint capsule)

anatomical structures of the infant's hip very well. However, it is not suitable for routine and especially not for preliminary diagnosis.

1.4.3 Magnetic Resonance Imaging (MRI)

Magnetic resonance imaging (MRI) provides excellent images and, depending on the machine and the slice thickness, demonstrates the fine

Learning point
MRI has its place in particularly difficult cases to assess the position of the hip joint in the socket and to evaluate successful reduction.

1.4.4 Ultrasonography

The Discovery of Ultrasound

One would assume that nocturnal animals have large eyes and exceptionally good eyesight, but in the case of bats, the opposite is true: they have strikingly small eyes but very large ears. This led the Italian researcher Spalanzani to conduct some experiments on the orientation ability of bats almost 200 years ago. He stretched thin threads with bells across a room, darkened the room, and let some bats fly around in it. Despite the complete darkness, none of the bats collided with the stretched threads. However, when their ears were plugged, they frequently touched the threads and even collided into the walls. Spalanzani's research laid the groundwork for the understanding that bats navigate in the dark through the ultrasound waves they emit, using the system of echolocation.

Technical Applications

The discovery of the piezoelectric effect in 1880 by the Curie brothers led to ultrasound waves being generated for the first time. The first practical system of echolocation was developed by A. von Sternbert, which opened up wide marine applications for ultrasound following the Titanic disaster in 1912. Some examples of the non-medical use of ultrasound include marine geology for measuring depths in the ocean or locating fish shoals. During the First World War, ultrasound was further developed by French physicist P. Langevin for military purposes, specifically for locating submarines. These applications demonstrate the versatility of ultrasound technology in various fields, including medical diagnostics, marine geology, and military applications.

Medical Applications

The application of ultrasound in medicine was introduced by the neurologist K. Th. Dussik in 1938. He and his brother, a radio technician, conducted initial experiments to show pathological changes in the skull using ultrasound. However, these experiments did not lead to a breakthrough in the use of ultrasound technology in medicine. It was not until 1954, with the introduction of a new generation of ultrasound machines with a water bath by J. G. Holmes, that a new milestone was reached. The studies by cardiologists J. Edler and C. H. Hertz on the heart caused a sensation in the medical world and led to the establishment of echocardiography. The subsequent rapid development culminated in a scanner developed by J. Donald and T. E. Braun without a water bath, providing two-dimensional imaging of almost all organs in the abdomen, as well as the heart and thyroid.

The History of Hip Ultrasound

Inspired by the findings of Kramps and Lenschow in 1978, the author and his team started systematically exploring possible applications of ultrasound in the musculoskeletal system. Encouraged by the results of muscle and tendon examinations, they also explored the use of ultrasound in infant hips, which initially yielded frustrating results due to an unexpected interplay of echo-poor and echo-rich areas. To understand these results better, they experimented with cadaveric hips, where they added reflective markers (Kolophonium, Metallic markers) to specific structures in order to identify them in the sonogram.

Through meticulous comparison of sonograms with cadaveric preparations, X-rays, arthrograms, hip joint sections, and cadaveric images in the form of diaphanograms, they gradually improved the understanding and identification of anatomical structures in the sonogram. Comparison series of sonograms of dislocated and non-dislocated hip joints revealed different but consistent echo patterns.

At that time, being mainly focused on X-ray images, they concentrated on the sonographic echoes of bone contours and the changes in their shape depending on the position of the femoral head. This technique allowed for the basic differentiation between dislocated and centred hips [22]. A milestone was reached when the ultrasound machine, borrowed from a friend, and the materials paid for out of the authors' own pocket, were replaced by an official research grant from the Austrian Science Fund. The idea of being able to detect the so-called congenital hip dislocation right after birth, without an X-ray, was almost unbelievable and was doubted and ridiculed by many colleagues. The classification of the different appearances of the cartilaginous acetabulum in healthy and pathological hip joints led to the realization that there is a wide variation between healthy and pathological.

The term "dislocated" had to be divided into several subtypes, including the term physiologically immature, which was responsible for some astonishing treatment success stories. Interestingly, it was an orthopaedic doctor from Bamberg, Dr. Röhr, who, after reading the first publication [22], wanted to be trained in the use of this technique, which at the time was still quite basic. Thanks to K. Rossak and his former student P. Schuler (St. Vincenz Hospital, Karlsruhe), hip sonography first sparked interest and made its way into the clinical field. K. Rossak deserves credit as a mentor for tirelessly driving hip sonography forward in Germany. P. Schuler critically reviewed the scientific findings for their accuracy and organized the first training courses in Germany for interested doctors.

The technique itself has evolved over the years, as evidenced by the gradual expansion of hip types. Expectations around the precision of the ultrasound technique have continually increased, leading to further developments and innovations, such as the clarification of the echoes of the proximal perichondrium [23] due to improved resolution. When the significance of tilting errors was recognized [24], an ultrasound probe guide apparatus was developed to avoid them.

> **Learning Points**
> Hip sonography was introduced as a screening method for all newborn hips in Austria in 1992, in Germany in 1996, in Switzerland in 1997, and in Mongolia in 2015 (with restrictions). In many countries, limited or selective hip ultrasound screening is carried out depending on the individual local healthcare systems.

1.5   The Current State of Hip Sonography Worldwide

Hip dysplasia is one of the commonest musculoskeletal pathologies, with an incidence of 2–4%.

Worldwide hip dysplasia remains the commonest cause of early hip osteoarthritis, leading to early total hip joint replacement in young adults [25], causing significant suffering for those affected (Fig. 1.3). The consensus worldwide is that treatment should be initiated promptly in early childhood, as late detection is associated with the need for more invasive treatment, a higher rate of complications, and worse treatment outcomes [26].

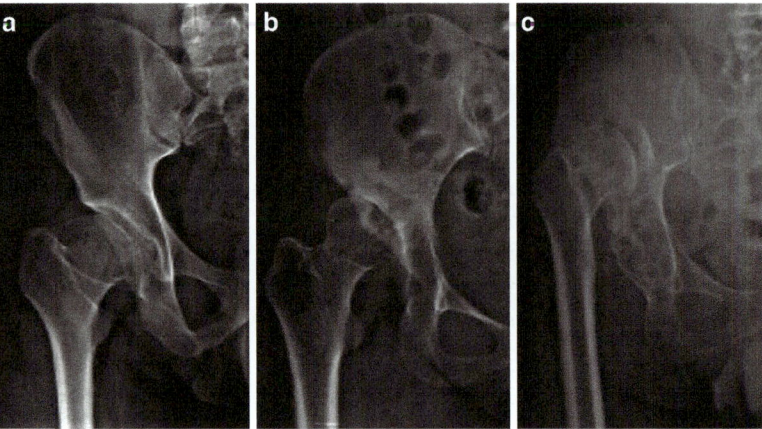

Fig. 1.3 Long-term outcome of a hip dislocation (**a**) coxa vara following femoral head necrosis (**b**) hip arthritis due to acetabular dysplasia (**c**) persistent high hip dislocation

1.5.1   Current Problems

Hip dysplasia is still approached with a wide range of diagnostic tests, including clinical examination, X-ray imaging, and ultrasound examination of the hip. Ultrasound is basically a dynamic examination so a standard plane has been defined to ensure reproducibility and comparability. The examination technique also allows for the so-called stress test if needed. As stated above, clinical examination alone cannot solve the problem of early diagnosis as it cannot detect mild dysplasia, which only becomes symptomatic once osteoarthritis develops, sometimes even in young adulthood [27–30]. Therefore, clinical examination alone is considered unreliable [31]. X-rays were considered the gold standard for the diagnosis of DDH until the 1980s.

Learning points
The unreliability of the interpretation of X-ray images due to only partial ossification of the hip in newborns plus the radiation exposure prohibit the use of X-rays for screening.

To better show the relationship between the femoral head and acetabulum and thus detect a possible disorder of hip maturation early, ultrasound examination is the most appropriate method for diagnosis in early infancy. This fact, together with the current consensus on the need for the earliest possible treatment of DDH, means that ultrasound examination of the hip joint should, without doubt, be the diagnostic test of choice.

Although the method is now established in many countries throughout the world to avoid radiation exposure, modifications of the technique have led to further disagreement and discussion. There is also debate about the best timing for US examination.

1.5.2   Examination Techniques

After its initial publication [22], ultrasound examination of infant hips became popular in the 1980s. Other ultrasound examination techniques include those developed by Harcke, Terjesen, and Suzuki. There are significant differences in their execution and interpretation:

- The Graf method, exclusively uses a linear ultrasound probe and requires a strictly lateral position of the infant during the examination. The sonogram can only be measured and interpreted after certain anatomical structures have been correctly identified and a usability check has been performed. The method is therefore strictly standardized. Both static and dynamic examinations are possible. When appropriate, a dynamic examination can be performed in addition to producing a standardised, static image
- Theodor Harcke developed his method in 1984 in the USA [32]. The positioning of the infant is variable, allowing for positioning either on the back or side. Four standard planes are possible but not mandatory. The combination of two perpendicular planes is used for the diagnosis, measuring the percentage coverage of the femoral head.
- Terje Terjesen established his method in the late 1980s in Norway [33]. Either a linear or a sector probe can be used. Both the frontal and transverse planes are examined statically and dynamically. A numerical measurement and a descriptive interpretation then leads to the diagnosis.
- Suzuki developed his method in the late 1980s in Japan [34]. The hip is scanned from anterior with a linear ultrasound probe while the baby is lying on its back. A standard plane is set for measurement. If a dislocated hip is suspected, an additional examination in a modified position must be performed.

The last three methods cited were not able to establish themselves for general screening for various reasons or were abandoned, as happened in Japan.

1.5.3   Screening

Despite the relatively high incidence of DDH and its potentially severe sequelae, there is currently no clear, internationally uniform guideline for the implementation and timing of a diagnostic examination. Selective ultrasound screening is advocated in many places especially for example, in English speaking and Scandinavian countries. This approach involves initially conducting a clinical examination on all babies, with an ultrasound examination of the hip only being performed if there are abnormalities in the clinical examination or if there are pre-existing risk factors. This approach carries the risk that many, especially mild, hip maturation disorders may not be detected and could cause early onset osteoarthritis in these patients [37].

The fact that general hip ultrasound screening in infancy has been introduced in only a few European and Asian countries, despite evidence showing a significant decrease in the number of surgical interventions following the introduction of hip ultrasound screening, seems surprising [38–44]. This decrease not only benefits the affected patients but also has socio-economic advantages. Regional US screening is established in China, Iran, Oman, Israel, Chile, and many other countries. In general, the policy on hip US screening is a political decision and depends on the organization of the local healthcare system. The public health system is publicly funded, and cost must be controlled. Hip US screening can help reduce the overall cost for the health system. This has already been statistically proven, especially in Austria, where general US screening was introduced over 30 years ago [40, 44, 45]. Austria is a relatively small country, and the number of children affected and those who are operated on can easily be captured, which makes the statistical analysis relatively easy and accurate. A significant reduction of surgical intervention for DDH, such as pelvic osteotomies in childhood, as well as total hip replacement surgery for young adults, was achieved and documented [38, 40]. The introduction of hip screening not only has positive financial implications but also reduces the need for various operations and hospital stays for children with hip dysplasia. This benefits not only the children but also their parents, who would otherwise have to take time off work and organize sick or carers leave to care for their hospitalized child. The time off needed for each affected child can be weeks to months, and the overall burden of cost is on the individual but ultimately on the welfare system and public funds.

For patients who have already joined the workforce—many professions are not compatible with hip dysplasia—symptomatic hip dysplasia and osteoarthritis of the hip can cause a great deal of personal suffering. Affected individuals experience daily life that is eventually characterized by pain and functional limitations, as well as having a limping, "waddling" gait, which can be seen as a stigma in our otherwise perfect world.

General hip ultrasound screening, therefore, provides specific psychological, social, and economic benefits. Convinced of the benefits of early hip sonography, some other European countries have established national general hip ultrasound screening programmes (e.g. Hungary, the Czech Republic, and Poland). However, there are still opponents to general ultrasound screening. In the English-speaking countries, concerns have been raised about too many false-positive cases and over-treatment when using the Graf method [46]. It is important to refute these concerns, as the examination technique is standardized in its performance and provides clear appropriate treatment according to hip type. A clear distinction between an immature hip, a hip with delayed ossification, and a pathological hip can be made, and the appropriate treatment pathway is clearly defined.

As with any other medical condition, one needs to acquire the appropriate knowledge and to build competence with the diagnostic techniques and procedures and appropriate treatment pathways. In this context, the claim that the Graf hip types are too complicated must be clearly refuted, as the precise differentiation by description of hip types takes into account the full spectrum of hip dysplasia in its different severities.

Accurate knowledge of the condition and consistent application of the diagnostic technique, as demanded in any medical practice, also reduces the number of false-positive cases and the associated, often criticized over-treatment. Type IIa joints are physiologically immature, do not require treatment, and can be monitored.

Learning points

A general US screening programme, which has been shown to be effective and only requires relatively cheap equipment, is recommended for every healthcare system and every country.

References

1. Ortolani M. Un segno poco noto e sua importanze per la diagnosi precoce di prelussazione congenita dell' anca. Pediatria. 1937;45:129–36.
2. Von Rosen S. Die konservative Behandlung der Hüftdysplasie und Hüftverrenkung. Z Orthop. 1969;106:173–8.
3. Barlow TG. Early diagnosis and treatment of congenital dis- location of the hip. J Bone Joint Surg Br. 1962;44-B:292–301.
4. Becker F. Probleme und Gefahren der funktionellen Behandlung dysplastischer Hüftgelenke im frühen Säuglingsalter. Z Orthop. 1979;117:138–46.
5. Schultheiss H. Frühbehandlung der Hüftdysplasie durch atraumatische Spreizung. Z Orthop. 1965:100.
6. Ackermann HJ, Kupper H. Zum Krankheitswert des „atypical dry click" an der Neugeborenenhüfte Beitr Orthop Traumat 1984; 31: 105–107
7. von Rosen S. Prophylaxe, Frühdiagnostik und Frühbehand- lung der Luxationshüfte. Beitr Orthop Traumatol. 1977;24:257–64.
8. Weickert H. Fortschritte in der Diagnostik und Behandlung der Luxationshüfte. Pädiatrie. 1975;14:63–9.
9. Breninek A. Stumme Fälle von Hüftdysplasie. Z Orthop. 1979;117:821–3.
10. Tönnis D. Congenital dysplasia and dislocation of the hip in children and adults. Berlin: Springer; 1987.
11. Weil UH. Acetabular dysplasia – skeletal dysplasias in child- hood. Progress in orthopaedic surgery 2. Berlin: Springer; 1978.
12. Roser W. Die Lehre von den Spontanluxationen. Arch Physiol Heilk. 1864;5:132–42.
13. Heipertz W, Maronna U. Der Wert der Röntgenunter- suchung in den ersten sechs Lebenswochen. In: Fries G, Tönnis D, editors. Hüftluxation und Hüftdysplasie. Uelzen: Med Lit Verlag; 1982. p. 25–9.
14. Tönnis D. Die angeborene Hüftdysplasie und Hüftluxation im Kindes- und Erwachsenenalter. Berlin: Springer; 1984.
15. Werzinger RA. Die kongenitale Hüftluxation. In: Konservative und operative Therapie [Dissertation]. München: Universität München; 1989.
16. Witt HJ, Woltersdorf J. Zwillingsuntersuchungen zur Luxationshüfte [Dissertation]. Magdeburg: Universität Magde- burg; 1986.
17. Büschelberger H. Die Luxationshüfte. In: Matzen P, editor. Lehrbuch der Orthopädie. Berlin: Volk und Gesundheit; 1982.
18. Faber A. Untersuchungen über die Ätiologie und Pathogenese der angeborenen Hüftverrenkung. Leipzig: Thieme; 1938.
19. Niethard FU, Gärtner BM. Die prognostische Bedeutung qualitativer Hüftparameter bei der Verlaufsbeobachtung der Hüftdysplasie im Säuglingsalter und Kleinkindesalter. In: Fries G, Tönnis D, editors. Hüftluxation und Hüftdysplasie. Uelzen: Med Lit Verlag; 1982. p. 56–9.

20. Peic S. Technische Erleichterung für die Durchführung einer Hüftarthrographie und Verhinderung der Entstehung der Wabenstruktur im Arthrogramm. In: Fries G, Tönnis D, editors. Hüftluxation und Hüftdysplasie. Uelzen: Med Lit Verlag; 1981. p. 71–4. atraumatische Spreizung. Z Orthop 1965; 100.

21. Schwetlick W. Die kindliche Luxationshüfte. Stuttgart: En- ke; 1976.

22. Graf R. The diagnosis of congenital hip joint dislocation by the ultrasonic compound treatment. Arch Orthop Traumat. 1980;97:117–33.

23. Graf R, Fronhöfer G. Neudefinition des proximalen Perichondriums und des Perichondriumloches im Hüftsonogramm. Orthopade. 1997;26:1057–61.

24. Graf R. Hüftsonographie. Grundsätze und aktuelle Aspekte. Orthopade. 1997;26:14–24.

25. Engesæter IØ, Lehmann T, Laborie LB, et al. Total hip re- placement in young adults with hip dysplasia: age at diagnosis, previous treatment, quality of life, and validation of diagnoses reported to the Norwegian Arthroplasty Register between 1987 and 2007. Acta Orthop. 2011;82(2):149–5.

26. Mulpuri K, Song KM, Goldberg MJ, et al. Detection and non- operative management of pediatric developmental dysplasia of the hip in infants up to six months of age. J Am Acad Orthop Surg. 2015;23(3):202–5.

27. Furnes O, Lie SA, Espehaug B, et al. Hip disease and the prognosis of total hip replacements. A review of 53 698 primary total hip replacements reported to the Norwegian Arthroplasty Register 1987–99. J Bone Joint Surg Br. 2001;83(4):579–86.

28. Holen KJ, Tegnander A, Bredland T, et al. Universal or selective screening of the neonatal hip using ultrasound? A prospective, randomised trial of 15 529 newborn infants. J Bone Joint Surg Br. 2002;84(6):886–90.

29. Macnicol MF. Results of a 25-year screening programme for neonatal hip instability. J Bone Joint Surg Br. 1990;72(6):1057–60.

30. Rosendahl K, Markestad T, Lie RT. Ultrasound screening for developmental dysplasia of the hip in the neonate: the effect on treatment rate and prevalence of late cases. Pedia- trics. 1994;94:47–52.

31. O'Beirne JG, Chlapoutakis K, Alshryda S, et al. International interdisciplinary consensus meeting on the evaluation of developmental dysplasia of the hip. Ultraschall Med. 2019;40(4):454–6.

32. Harcke HT, Clarke NMP, Lee MS, et al. Examination of the infant hip with real-time ultrasonography. J Ultrasound Med. 1984;3:131–7.

33. Terjesen T, Rundén TO, Tangerud A. Ultrasonography and radiography of the hip in infants. Acta Orthop Scand. 1989;60(6):651–60.

34. Suzuki S, Awaya G, Wakita S, et al. Diagnosis by ultrasound of congenital dislocation of the hip joint. Clin Orthop. 1987;217:172–8.

35. Roovers EA, Boere-Boonekamp MM, Geertsma TSA, et al. Ultrasonographic screening for developmental dysplasia of the hip in infants. Reproducibility of assessments made by radiographers. J Bone Joint Surg Br. 2003;85:726–30.

36. Simon EA, Saur F, Buerge M, et al. Inter-observer agreement of ultrasonographic measurement of alpha and beta angles and the final type classification based on the Graf method. Swiss Med Wkly. 2004;134(45–46):671–7.

37. Sink EL, Ricciardi BF, Torre K, et al. Selective ultrasound screening is inadequate to identify patients who present with symptomatic adult acetabular dysplasia. J Child Orthop. 2014;8(6):451–5.

38. Biedermann R, Riccabona J, Giesinger JM, et al. Results of universal ultrasound screening for developmental dysplasia of the hip: a prospective follow-up of 28 092 consecutive infants. J Bone Joint Surg Br. 2018;100-B(10):1399–404.

39. Ganger R, Grill F, Leodolter S, et al. Ultraschall-Screening der Neugeborenenhüfte: Ergebnisse und Erfahrungen. Ultraschall Med. 1991;12:25–30.

40. Grill F, Müller D. Ergebnisse des Hüftultraschallscreenings in Österreich. Orthopade. 1997;26:25–32.

41. von Kries R, Ihme N, Oberle D, et al. Effect of ultrasound screening on the rate of first operative procedures for developmental hip dysplasia in Germany. Lancet. 2003;362:1883–7.

42. von Kries R, Ihme N, Altenhofen L, et al. General ultrasound screening reduces the rate of first operative procedures for developmental dysplasia of the hip: a case-control study. J Pediatr. 2012;160(2):271–5.

43. Thallinger C, Pospischill R, Ganger R, et al. Long-term results of a nationwide general ultrasound screening system for developmental disorders of the hip: the Austrian hip screening program. J Child Orthop. 2014;8:3–10.

44. Tschauner C, Furntrath F, Saba Y, et al. Developmental dysplasia of the hip: impact of sonographic newborn hip screening on the outcome of early treated decentered hip joints – a single center retrospective comparative cohort study based on Graf's method of hip ultrasonography. J Child Orthop. 2011;5:415–24.

45. Ashraf A, Larson AN, Maradit-Kremers H, et al. Hospital costs of total hip arthroplasty for developmental dysplasia of the hip. Clin Orthop Relat Res. 2014;472(7):2237–44.

46. Paton RW. Screening in developmental dysplasia of the hip (DDH). Surgeon. 2017;15(5):290–6.

Hip Ultrasound Technique, Equipment, and Image Projection

2

The scientific principles have been described in detail and are widely recognized [1].

2.1 Equipment

2.1.1 Transducer

Types of Transducers

The compound scanners that were originally used have been replaced by high-resolution real-time scanners—be it sector, trapezoidal, or linear ultrasound transducers.

Since both sector and linear transducers have their advantages and disadvantages, depending on the field of application, the selection of the appropriate transducer is based on the anatomical area to be examined. For instance, meniscus sonography largely provides satisfactory results with sector transducers, while for the shoulder joint, sector and linear transducers as well as curved array transducers are in use.

The ability to show movements through real-time scanners is particularly invaluable in what are known as dynamic or stress examinations.

The curved array transducer attempts to balance the advantages and disadvantages of sector and linear transducers as a "compromise transducer". It should not be used for the diagnosis of disorders of hip maturation because of the risk of diffraction or refraction artefacts due to the obliquity of the incoming sound waves.

▶ **Tip** It cannot be emphasized enough that the choice of transducer fundamentally depends on the organ to be examined. A linear transducer must be used for the infant hip.

Sector Versus Linear Transducer for the Sonographic Diagnosis of Hip Dysplasia

A critical comparison of the advantages and disadvantages of linear and sector transducers in hip sonography was conducted by K. Schneider [2]. Based on studies and calculations [3], it must be expressly stated that when ultrasound beams are not parallel on entry, there is significant potential for distortion due to diffraction and refraction artefacts, resulting in incorrect angle values. Theoretical calculations on a computer model confirm the clinical experience that the significant potential for distortion can affect the quality of the hip sonogram when the transducer is tilted, leading to obliquely angled ultrasound waves (p. 67) imaging the hip joint.

> Caution: Hip ultrasonography requires an ultrasound beam that enters perpendicular and parallel to the body axis. With obliquely incoming sound waves, the different sound propagation speeds in muscle, cartilage, and bone, lead to distortions according to Snellius's law of refraction. These potential distortions can lead to misdiagnosis.

According to more recent studies, a trapezoidal transducer appears to be equivalent to a linear transducer because it also emits waves that largely run parallel to each other.

2.1.2 Device Settings and Frequencies

Device Settings

The most important variables for machine settings are:

- the sound intensity or gain
- the focal depth
- the contrast
- pre- and post-processing

> Note: Without going into details, the ultrasound machine should be set so that the hyaline cartilage and femoral head appear hypoechoic not anechoic.

Frequencies

Frequency and depth of penetration are inversely proportional to each other: as the frequency increases, the resolution improves while the depth of penetration decreases, and vice versa. Therefore, the hip joints of newborns with their small anatomical structures at shal-

low depths are appropriately examined using frequencies of 7.0 or 7.5 MHz and higher. Larger children, whose hip joints cannot be fully imaged using a 7-MHz probe due to inadequate depth penetration, especially for displaying critical structures such as the lower limb of the os ilium, should be examined with a 5-MHz transducer.

2.1.3 Hip Sonography-Specific Equipment

The hip joint should always be examined under standardized conditions. It is necessary to minimize problems caused by the child's natural leg movements as well as by the examiners themselves. This has led to the development of a very specific handling technique during the examination (see p. 59). Also to the development of a cradle and ultrasound probe guide system to prevent tilting errors, which can lead to misdiagnosis (see Fig. 2.1). Cradle and probe guide are a

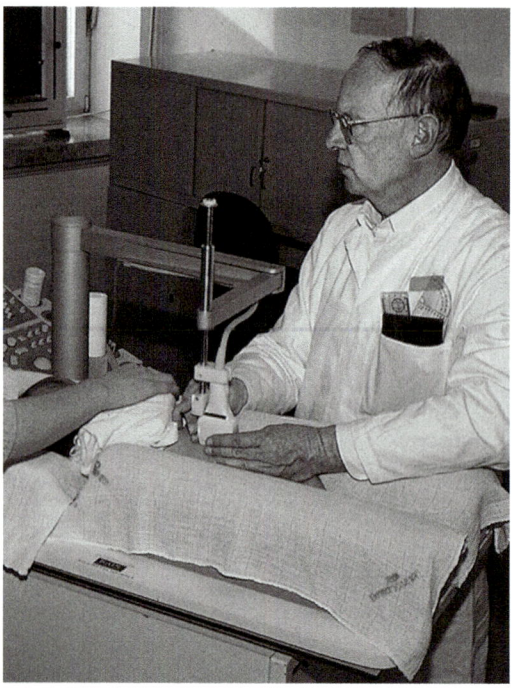

Fig. 2.1 Ultrasound probe guide to prevent tilting errors

mandatory requirement to fulfil the modern high standards of the examination technique.

> **Note**
> Never perform freehand scanning of the infant hip

The ultrasound gel can be stored at room temperature. Warming of the gel is usually not necessary if the correct scanning technique is used, especially as the gel can become runnier (lower viscosity) when warmed, and its sound-conducting properties may deteriorate.

Buttons to freeze the image directly on the transducer or a footswitch are strongly recommended. Freeze buttons only on the ultrasound machine itself are often inadequate as operating the transducer with one hand usually results in the loss of the standard plane. The magnification function should be high performance. The scale depicted on the US picture or printout must be at least 1.7: 1.

Most US machines can, at the push of a button, rotate the horizontal projection (abdominal sonography) into the vertical right hip projection. The electronic measurement of alpha and beta angles on the screen significantly simplifies the documentation in routine practice.

A semi-automatic scanning process, independent of the examiner's skill level and with a high standard of precision, has been developed and will soon be ready for use in routine practice.

▶ **Practical tip Required equipment for hip US:**
- cradle
- probe guide system
- gel (ready to use)
- transducer with 5+ MHz

2.2   Documentation

In principle, a descriptive report and a hip sonogram with the corresponding morphological findings must be available. The importance of the morphological description will be explained later (p. 94). With regard to the requirements for the hip sonogram itself, we have to distinguish between formal and methodological image criteria.

2.2.1   Standard Image Criteria

Picture scale
The image scale must not be less than 1.7:1. This minimum scale is necessary to provide clarity of important image details. Additionally, the size of the image should allow for the manual measurement of printed sonograms. The same applies to digitally stored images.

Anatomical projection of hip sonograms and the right-sided projection
All hip sonograms, regardless of whether they are of the right or left hip, are projected so that they resemble a right anteroposterior hip X-ray image (anatomical projection). Our studies have shown that right-sided projections of an erect hip joint, showed diagnostic error rates that were one-third lower than for those projected to the left (see Fig. 2.2).

The reason why it is easier to see and interpret hip sonograms that are projected as though an erect AP view of a right hip, is neurophysiological and was vividly described by E. P. Fischer [2]. The phenomenon is based on the hemispheric dominance of one side of the brain. In recording eye movements during the inspection of a person by an observer, Engelen was able to demonstrate that the gaze almost exclusively concentrates on the right side of the body [3].

By consistently applying the same right projection to all hip sonograms, the examiner always achieves the same impression of the image. Slight changes in the coverage conditions and positional changes of the femoral head are thus recognized much more easily.

2.2.2   Methodological Image Criteria

(Documentation Guidelines)
The sonograms must fulfil the conditions of Checklist I (p. 46) and Checklist II (p. 49) (Fig. 2.3)

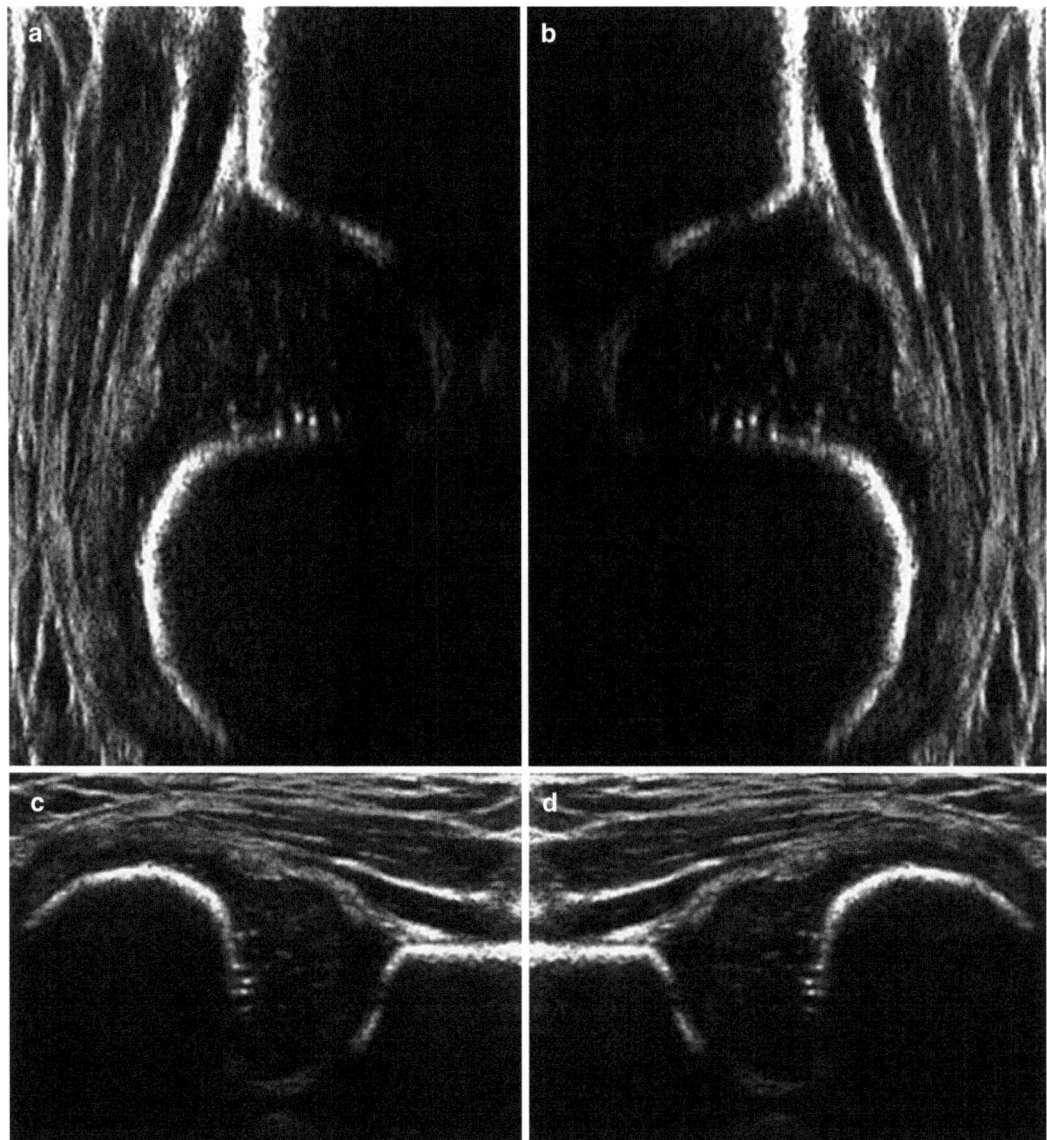

Fig. 2.2 Anatomical projections. Options for imaging projection. Projections such as b and d should be avoided in the diagnosis of DDH (**a**) Optimal erect right projection. Projection similar to a right hip joint in an anteropos- terior X-ray image (**b**) Inappropriate erect left projection (**c**) Alternative cranial right projection (**d**) Inappropriate cranial left projection

Due to the cross-sectional technique, for safety reasons, it is essential to document 2, time-staggered, sections of each hip according to the criteria mentioned above: the image conditions are not the same every time. Through a slight change of the reflection angle, individual details, such as the labrum, can often be better seen in other sections. One sonogram in the standard plane of a hip joint should be measured, whereas a second sonogram of the same hip joint should be saved without measurement lines to avoid covering up important reference points.

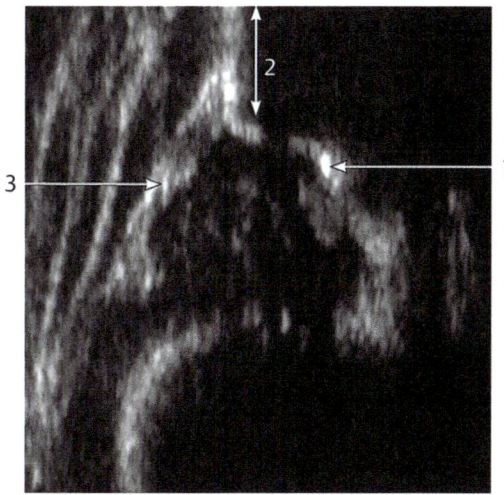

Fig. 2.3 Correct sonogram with the three landmarks of Checklist II. The points of Checklist I were not marked in this image. (1 = lower limb of the os ilium, 2 = straight echo of the iliac bone (plane), 3 = labrum)

▶ **Practical tip** Documentation: Save two separate images per hip joint in the standard plane, one of them with measurement lines indicating the α and β angles

- Image scale 1.7:1
- Erect right projection

References

1. Müller W. Biophysikalische Messungen zum Effekt von Kippfehlern bei der Hüftsonographie [mündliche Mitteilung]. 1998
2. Fischer EP. Die Welt im Kopf. Konstanz: Faude; 1985.
3. Engelen H. Die Evolution der Liebe. GEO. 1997;1:34–6.

Learning point
It is not sufficient to document a hip joint with only one image.

The Pillars of Hip Sonography

3

3.1 Development of the Hip Joint

Between the sixth and seventh week of gestation, the cartilaginous precursors of the three pelvic bones have merged into a single cartilaginous hemipelvis and form the shallow acetabulum. Between the acetabulum and the cartilaginous precursor of the femoral head, the future joint space is still filled with connective tissue. At this stage, the labrum can already be seen as increased density within the connective tissue [1]. In the seventh week, the early joint cavity, the ligamentum teres, and the joint capsule begin to form. By the end of the eighth week, the early development of the hip joint is already complete (see Fig. 3.1) [1, 2].

The femoral shaft starts to ossify as early as the seventh week of embryonic development, forming a bony tube and a central marrow cavity. By the end of the twelfth week of gestation, the femoral shaft ossification is complete.

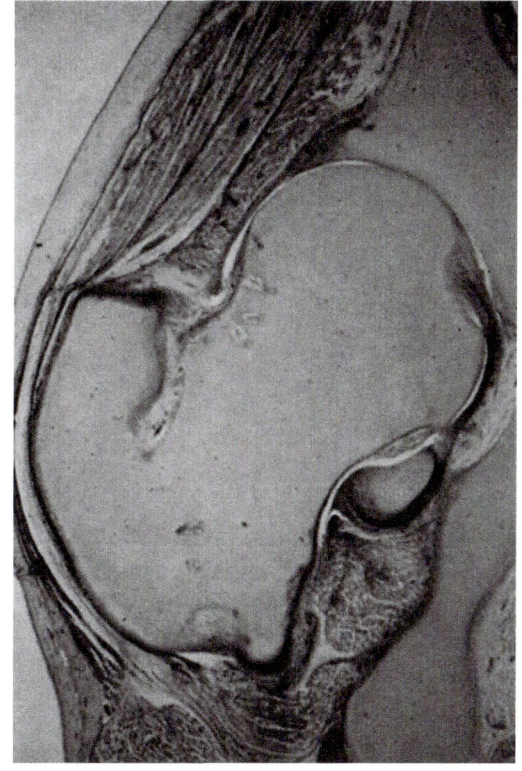

Fig. 3.1 Cross-section through an embryonic hip joint

R. Graf et al., *Sonography of the Infant's Hip*, https://doi.org/10.1007/978-3-031-71949-3_3

3.2   Direction of the Ultrasound Beam and the Soft Tissue Overlying the Hip

For the diagnosis of hip dysplasia and dislocation, the coronal plane through the hip joint is the only recommended plane with the current standard of the technique. This approach produces ultrasound images that correspond to an anatomical coronal section through the hip joint (see Figs. 3.2 and 3.3). In Fig. 3.4, the ultrasound penetrates from lateral to medial, first passing through the skin, then the subcutaneous tissue, the fascia lata, the gluteal muscles, and the intermuscular septa. The intermuscular septa are more echogenic than the surrounding muscles.

While it is possible to use different planes and scan for example from posterior or through the adductors with abducted legs (Lorenz position) [3], these other planes are not helpful in routine practice and do not provide additional useful information. The posterior imaging plane only allows for the visualization of completely dislocated femoral heads but does not provide information on potential deformity of the socket [4].

Examination techniques in the Lorenz position (anteroposterior beam direction), only show the anterior and posterior edges of the acetabular roof. However, pathological changes are found on the cranial or cranio-posterior part of the acetabular roof and are thus not assessed with this technique. The antero-posterior beam direction onto the femoral head in the Lorenz position allows for the sonographic measurement of the anteversion angle [5]. While it is possible to check the correct position of the femoral head with this plane after reducing a dislocated hip joint, the technical difficulties of the examination are significant, and quantification is difficult.

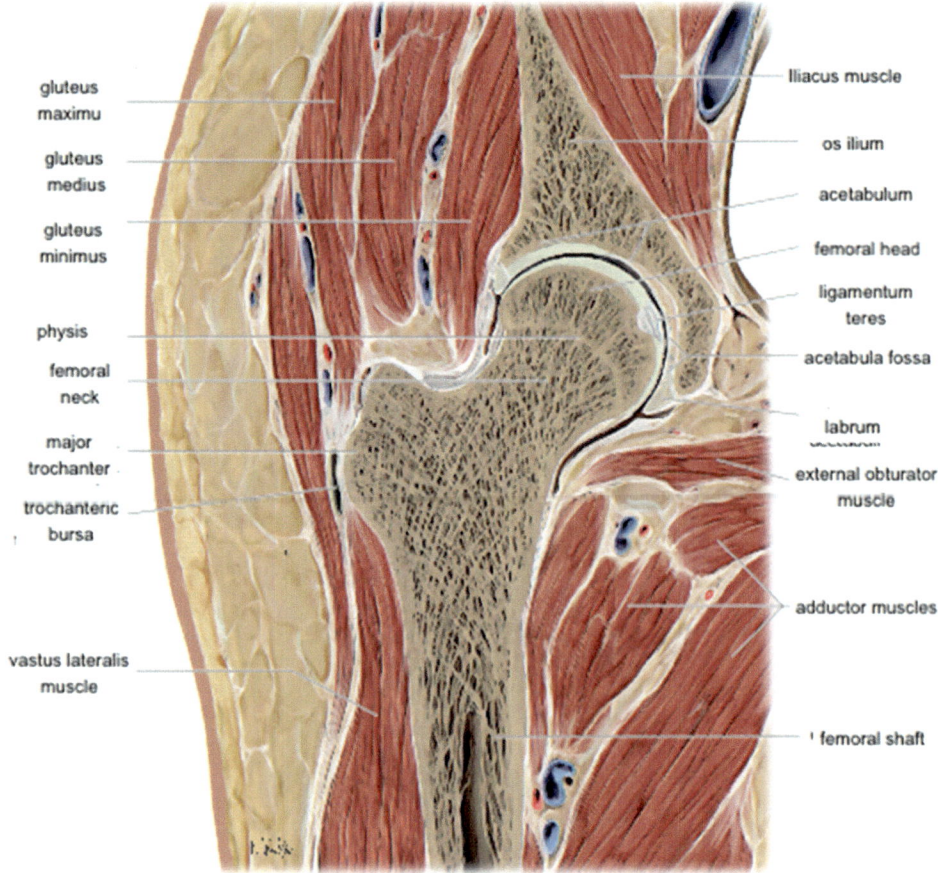

Fig. 3.2 Frontal section through a right hip joint. Schematic representation (Lig. = ligament, M./Mm. = muscle/muscles)

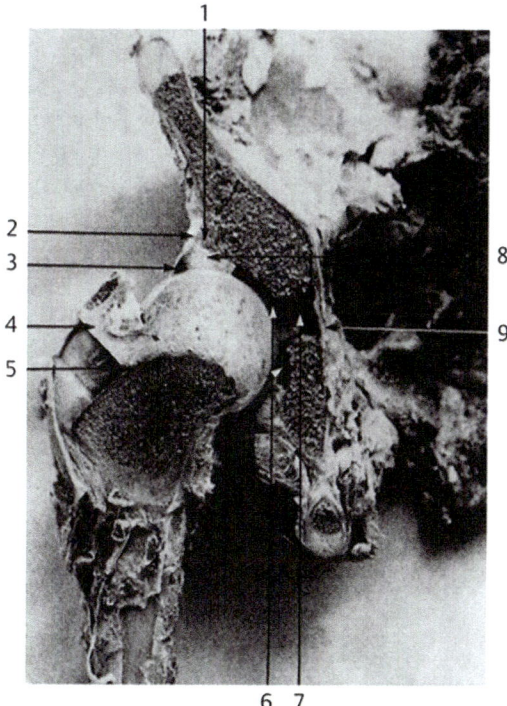

Fig. 3.3 Section of a child's hip joint (8 weeks old). Cf. Fig. 3.4 (1 = bony acetabular rim, 2 = perichondrium or periosteum of the ilium, 3 = labrum, 4 = greater trochanter, 5 = chondro-osseous border of the proximal femur, 6 = dissected acetabular fossa, 7 = dissected triradiate cartilage, 8 = cartilaginous acetabular roof, 9 = perichondrium on the inner wall of the pelvis)

3.3   Femoral Neck and Femoral Head

3.3.1   Anatomy and Development

The femoral head, the proximal part of the femoral neck, and the greater trochanter are all initially formed as hyaline cartilage (see Fig. 3.5). An ossification centre appears within the femoral head, and a second ossification centre is located in the greater trochanter. The timing of the appearance of the ossific nucleus in X-ray images is reported as variable: Putti speaks of a delayed appearance if the ossific nucleus is not visible until the third or fourth month of life [6]. Hilgenreiner states the average time of appearance is the fourth month [7]. According to Tönnis, pathological conditions should be considered if the ossific nuclei are not detectable in the second half of the first year of life [8].

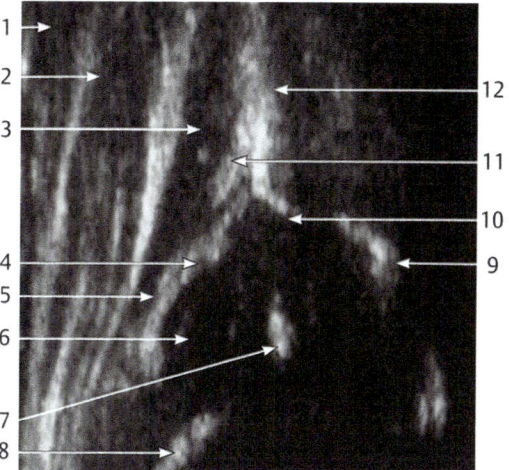

Fig. 3.4 Sonogram of a 3-month-old child (1 = gluteus maximus muscle, 2 = gluteus medius muscle, 3 = gluteus minimus muscle, 4 = labrum, 5 = joint capsule, 6 = femoral head, 7 = ossific nucleus of the femoral head, 8 = chondro-osseous border, 9 = lower limb of the ilium, 10 = bony acetabular rim, 11 = proximal perichondrium incl. Rectus tendon, 12 = iliac silhouette)

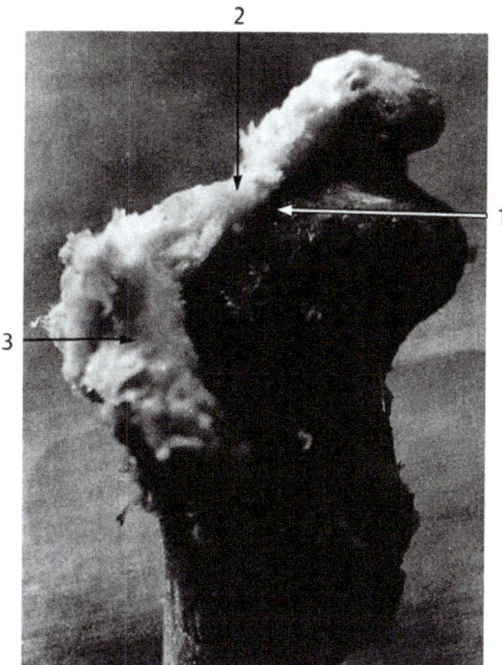

Fig. 3.5 Right proximal femur and ossific nucleus. The chondro-osseous border has been exposed, and the hyaline cartilage of the femoral neck and the base of the trochanter are clearly visible (1 = chondro-osseous border, 2 = hyaline cartilage of the femoral neck, 3 = base of the trochanter)

Note

As long as there are no ossific nuclei visible in the femoral head or the greater trochanter, the border between the cartilaginous and bony parts at the proximal end of the femur is referred to as the "chondro-osseous border".

3.3.2 Proximal Part of the Femur

After passing through the soft tissue mantle, the sound waves reach the proximal part of the femur.

The hyaline cartilage of the greater trochanter presents as a hypo-echogenic area and is peripherally delineated by the echoes of the tendon insertions into the trochanteric fossa and the greater trochanter (see Fig. 3.6). The chondro-osseous border, which is highly echogenic due to the total reflection of the sound beam by bone, divides the femoral neck into the proximal cap-like, hypoechoic portion that is hyaline cartilage, and into the distal bony portion, which gives an acoustic shadow. The chondro-osseous border is an important aid for orientation and for identification of the femoral neck and the femoral head.

With the current state of knowledge, the chondro-osseous border can also be instrumental in the recognition of tilting errors, which in some cases can lead to misdiagnoses, so it is strongly recommended to document it on a sonogram. Due to the varying growth potential of the medial and lateral ends of the chondro-osseous border, its shape also changes with age (see Fig. 3.7).

The age-dependent shape of the chondro-osseous border has sonographic significance:

- In new-borns, the chondro-osseous border still curves upward and can be followed deep into the acetabulum (see Fig. 3.8 and see Fig. 3.9).
- As the medial end of the chondro-osseous border becomes more angulated in the area between the head and the femoral neck in older infants (see Fig. 3.10), this part increasingly falls into the acoustic shadow. It can then often only be seen as parallel echo stripes described as palisades (see Fig. 3.11b and see Fig. 3.12).
- In still older infants, the medial part of the chondro-osseous border is even more angu-

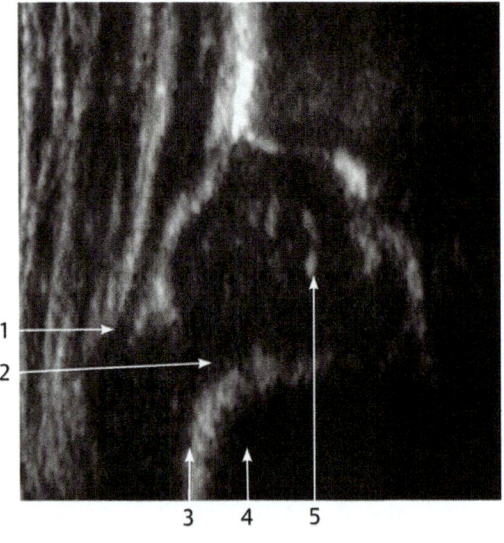

Fig. 3.6 Proximal femur in the sonogram (1 = trochanter with tendon attachment, 2 = hyaline cartilage of the femoral neck, 3 = chondro-osseous border, 4 = acoustic shadow behind the chondro-osseous border, 5 = femoral head (with sinusoids))

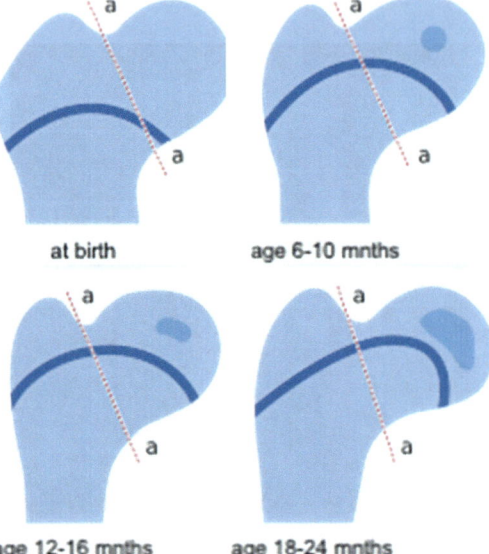

at birth   age 6-10 mnths

age 12-16 mnths   age 18-24 mnths

Fig. 3.7 Different appearances of the chondro-osseous border depending on age. Schematic representation [6] (**a**) attachment of the joint capsule

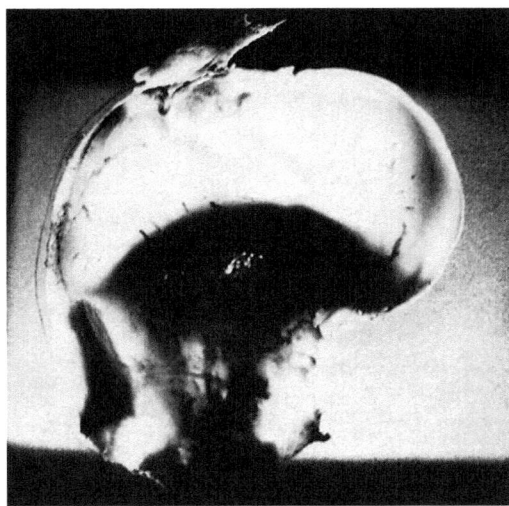

Fig. 3.8 Cadaveric diaphanogram image of the proximal part of the femur. The curved shape of the chondro-osseous border is visible

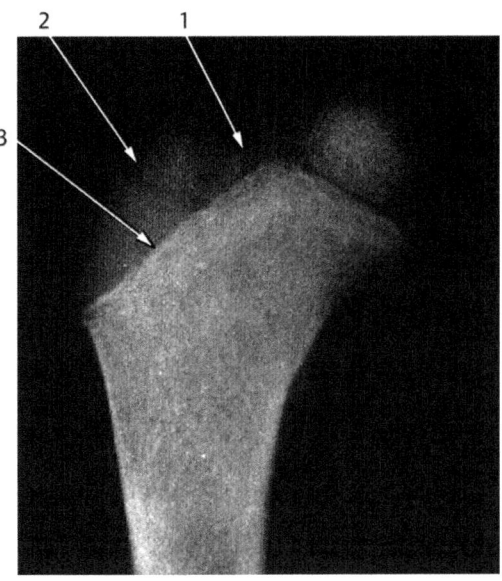

Fig. 3.10 X-ray image of the proximal end of the femur (1 = hyaline cartilage femoral neck 2 = greater trochanter, 3 = curved chondro-osseous border)

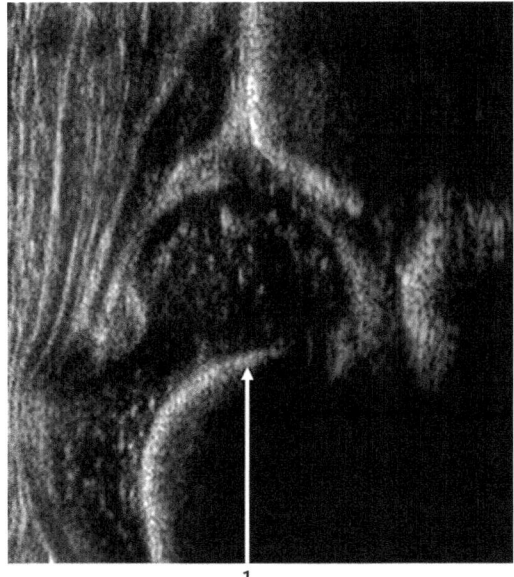

Fig. 3.9 Hip ultrasound of a newborn. The chondro-osseous border is clearly visible as an arc-like contour extending into the depth of the acetabular fossa (1 = chondro-osseous border)

lated and is completely in the acoustic shadow of the bony part of the femoral neck (see Fig. 3.13 and Fig. 3.10) and therefore is no longer visible. The visibility of the medial part of the chondro-osseous border also depends on the abduction or adduction of the femur. A summary of the possible echoes of the chondro-osseous border can be seen in Fig. 3.11.

3.3.3 Femoral Head and Ossific Nucleus

In the hyaline cartilage of the femoral head, small, dot-like echoes can be seen (see Fig. 3.14). They correspond to the sinusoids of the cartilage (see Fig. 3.15) that are also macroscopically visible in cross-sections (see Fig. 3.16). The sinusoids provide the blood supply to the femoral head and

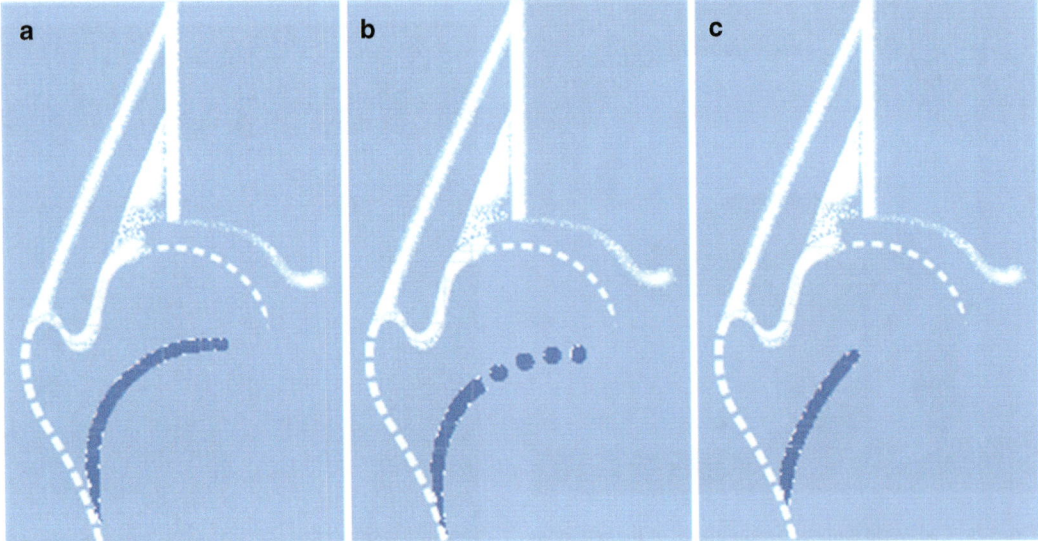

Fig. 3.11 Possible shapes of the chondro-osseous border (**a**) Arcuate, (**b**) Acoustic palisades, (**c**) Only the lateral part of the chondro-osseous border is visible

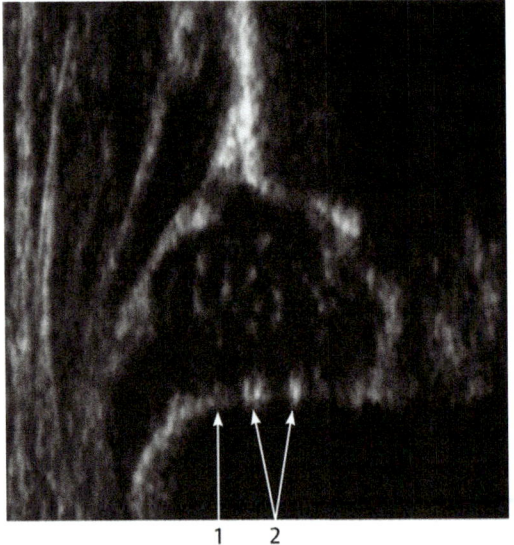

Fig. 3.12 Chondro-osseous border with the so-called sound palisades (1 = chondro-osseous border, 2 = sound palisades)

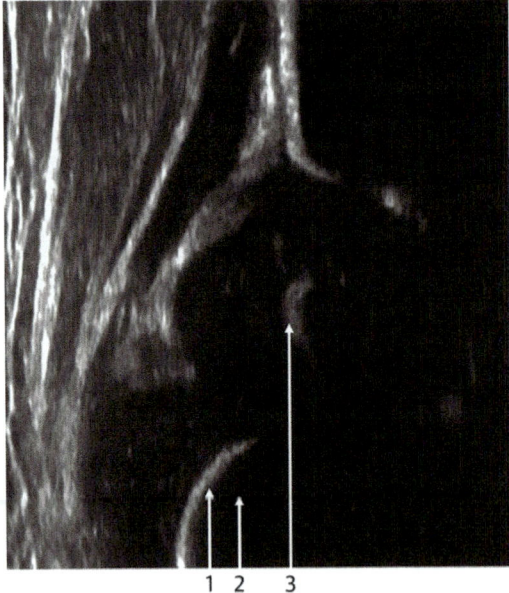

Fig. 3.13 Chondro-osseous border of an older infant. Only the lateral part of the chondro-osseous border is visible (1 = chondro-osseous border. 2 = acoustic shadow, 3 = femoral head ossific nucleus (half-moon phenomenon))

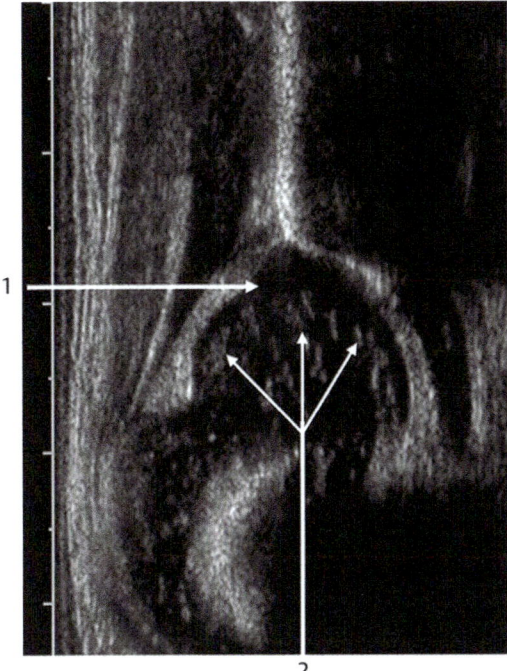

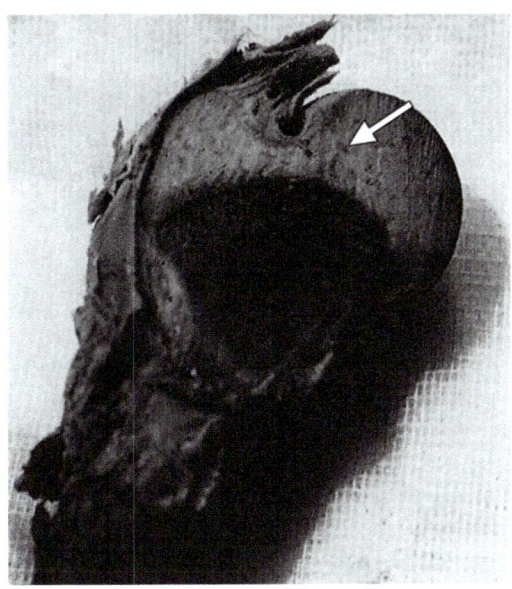

Fig. 3.16   Cross-section through the proximal end of the femur. The arcuate chondro-osseous border and the greater trochanter with tendon insertion are clearly visible, as are the sinusoids (arrow) in the hyaline cartilage

Fig. 3.14   Worm-like echoes in the hyaline portion of the femoral head. These echoes correspond to the sinusoids (1 = echo-poor marginal zone of the hyaline cartilage of the femoral head, (Annular zone) 2 = sinusoids (Central zone))

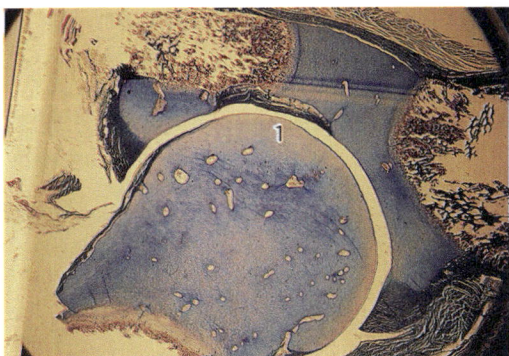

Fig. 3.15   Vascular sinusoids in the central zone. Histological cross section. The surface of the femoral head without recognizable sinusoids (1 = annular zone)

when compressed, can lead to femoral head necrosis. As the size of the cartilaginous parts increase with growth during the foetal period, diffusion alone is not sufficient for nourishment of the hyaline cartilage, and therefore temporary vascularization is provided from the perichondrium via blood-filled channels, the sinusoids [9].

Central Zone and Annular Zone

The surface of the femoral head has no sinusoids, and therefore appears on the sonogram as an annular hypoechoic zone (see Fig. 3.14). This annular zone is nourished by diffusion.

The author and his colleagues have referred to the sinusoid-free zone as the "Zona anularis" and the sinusoid-rich central zone as the "Zona centralis". The Zona anularis must not be confused with a hypoechoic hip joint effusion.

Geometry of the Femoral Head

> Learning point: One of the most essential and important points for hip ultrasound is the fact that the femoral head is not a sphere, but has a paraboloid shape (Pascal-paraboloid; nut or egg-shaped).

Accordingly, sections through the femoral head are not circles, but ovals that vary with the plane in which the hip has been depicted. This fact is crucial for the question of reproducibility of ultrasound images, as sections through the hip joint, since the image of the femoral head changes depending on the sonographic plane. For this reason, all the systems that include the centre of the femoral head in the measurements do not meet today's standards and have a high error rate potentially leading to misdiagnosis (e.g. "50% femoral head coverage by the acetabular roof") [10].

Ossific Nucleus

The ossific nucleus is not automatically located in the centre of the femoral head.

On ultrasound, the appearance of the ossific nucleus can be detected 4–8 weeks earlier than on an X-ray image. The reason for this is as follows:

During the formation of the ossification centre, from which further endochondral ossification of the epiphysis proceeds, mesenchymal cells are brought in through ingrowing perichondral vessels. These differentiate into osteoblasts and begin the production of osteoid. These tissue changes cause structural inhomogeneity which results in reflection of ultrasound waves during the initial formation of the ossific nucleus. Later, the mineralization of the newly formed osteoid occurs. Only then can the mineralized osteoid be recognized on an X-ray as an ossification centre.

A sonographic echo of the ossific nucleus can already be present at birth. The average age for the appearance of the nucleus in infants of normal maturity is 7.5 months.

Time Difference Between Sonographic Findings and X-Ray Image

The ossification processes can be seen in sonograms 4–6, in some cases even up to 8 weeks earlier than on an X-ray. This explains the discrepancy between an ultrasound image and an X-ray image taken at the same time. Anatomically, the ossific nucleus is not round but oval and is not automatically in the centre of the femoral head. For these two reasons, the ossific nucleus cannot be used to determine the position of the femoral head in relation to the acetabulum.

Sonographic Characteristics of the Ossific Nucleus

- **Half moon phenomenon** (see Fig. 3.17): With a large ossific nucleus and the sound

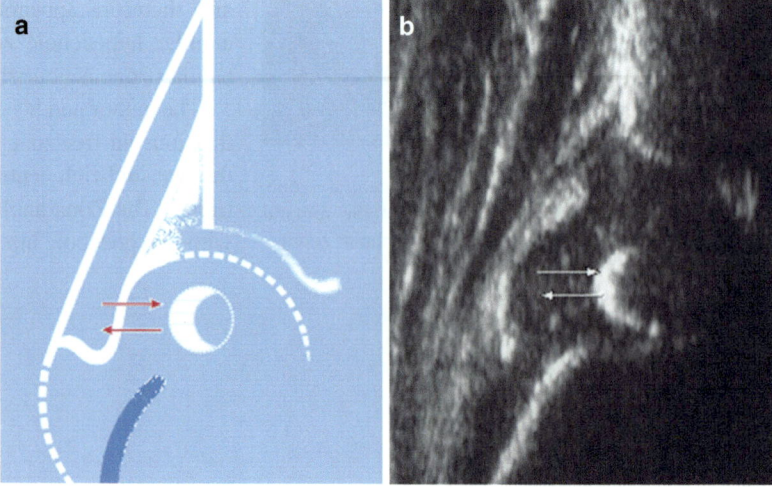

Fig. 3.17 Half-moon phenomenon (**a**) Due to complete reflection of US waves on bone creating an acoustic shadow, only the lateral portion of the ossific nucleus is visible. (**b**) Hip sonogram with clear crescent sign/halfmoon phenomenon (arrows)

waves coming from lateral the echoes are reflected by the lateral side of the ossific nucleus. The medial part of the ossific nucleus lies in the acoustic shadow of the lateral part. Therefore, a large ossific nucleus appears as a crescent-shaped echo in the sonogram.

- **Diagnostic error** (see Fig. 3.18): The ossific nucleus should not be used for diagnosis unlike in an X-ray image. The echo of the nucleus is not round and is not automatically in the centre of the femoral head. If one tries to determine the position of the head relative to the acetabulum, mistakenly using the Perkin's line and Hilgenreiner line as on an X-ray image, the ossific nucleus with only the lateral part visible as a crescent, suggests lateralization.
- **Size determination:** Since the ossific nucleus is not round and is not automatically the centre of the femoral head (compare Fig. 3.17b with Fig. 3.19), it cannot be predicted where the sound waves will hit the ossific nucleus. This depends on the position of the proximal part of the femur. If the sound waves hit the centre of the ossific nucleus, a large echo will be created.

If, on the other hand, the sound waves only hit the periphery of the ossific nucleus, only a small echo will be visible. A reproducible measurement of the size of the ossific nucleus in the sonogram is not possible.

- Limitation of the examination technique due to the ossific nucleus (see Fig. 3.20): The most important reference point in every hip sonogram is the lower limb of the os ilium in the acetabular fossa. If the lower limb of the os ilium is not visible, it is not certain that the plane goes through the centre of the acetabulum. If the lower limb of the os ilium is obscured by the acoustic shadow of a large ossific nucleus, the most important reference point of the sectional plane is missing. One exception is described later (p. 54).

If the degree of ossification of the femoral head causes the ossific nucleus to block the sound waves coming from lateral (see Fig. 3.20), and therefore the lower limb of the os ilium falls into the acoustic shadow of the ossific nucleus, ultrasound can no longer be used for diagnosis. The degree of ossification is the limiting factor to hip ultrasound, while age is only an indirect limitation.

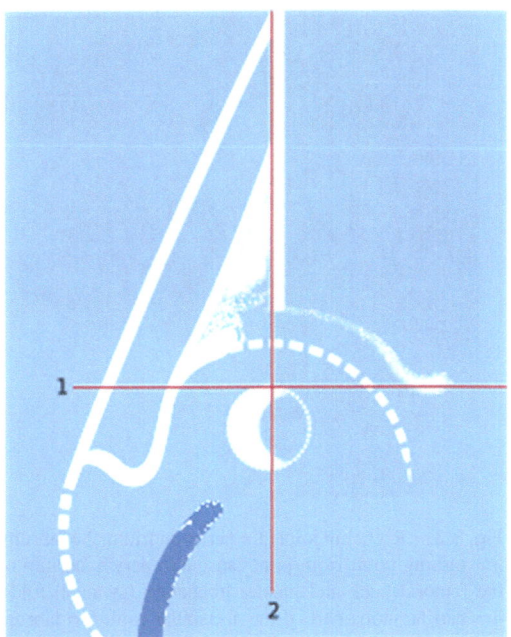

Fig. 3.18 Apparent lateralization or decentering caused by the crescent sign (1 = Hilgenreiner line, 2 = Perkins line)

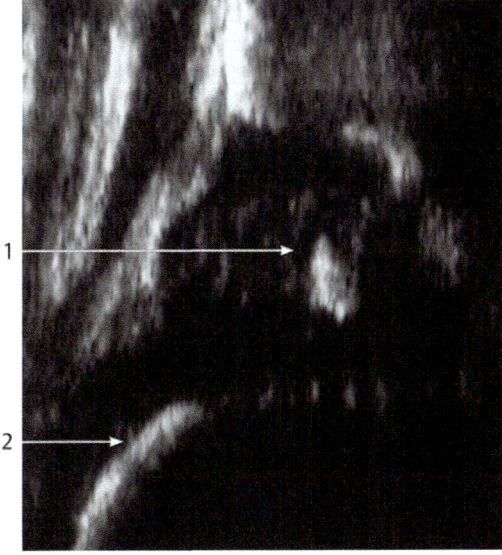

Fig. 3.19 Positional relationship of the ossific nucleus/femoral head. The ossific nucleus or its echo does not automatically lie in the centre of the femoral head (1 = nucleus, 2 = chondro-osseous border)

Fig. 3.20 Acoustic shadow of a large ossific nucleus (1 = ossific nucleus, 2 = acetabular labrum, 3 = bony rim) (**a**) Large ossific nucleus blocks the sound waves, so that the lower limb of the ilium falls into the acoustic shadow of the ossific nucleus. (**b**) The large ossific nucleus blocks the sound waves

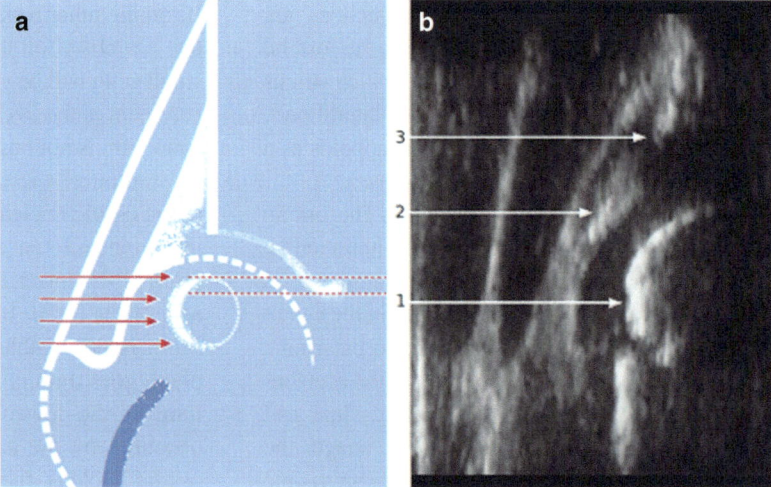

Conclusion

- The ossific nucleus is not the centre of the femoral head.
- It is not round.
- It must not be used as in X-rays for the diagnosis of a hip dislocation (crescent sign).
- It limits the technique (if the lower limb of the ilium is not visible).

3.3.4 Structures Surrounding the Femoral Head

The lateral side of the femoral head is adjacent to the joint capsule, which runs along the femoral neck and extends into the perichondrium of the greater trochanter in the area of the zona orbicularis (see Fig. 3.21).

Synovial Fold

In sonograms, where the joint capsule turns towards the periosteum of the femoral neck is called the synovial fold (see Fig. 3.22). It appears as an ill-defined echo or two parallel echo stripes. Following the synovial fold of the joint capsule upwards along the surface of the femoral head,

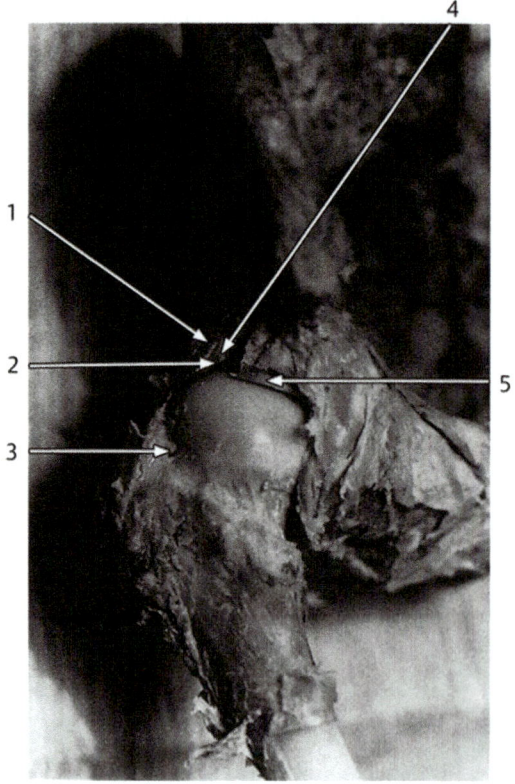

Fig. 3.21 Right hip joint (1 = perichondrium, 2 = labrum, 3 = turning point from joint capsule to perichondrium of the femoral neck and greater trochanter (synovial fold), 4 = cartilaginous part of the acetabular roof, 5 = labrum projecting freely into the joint)

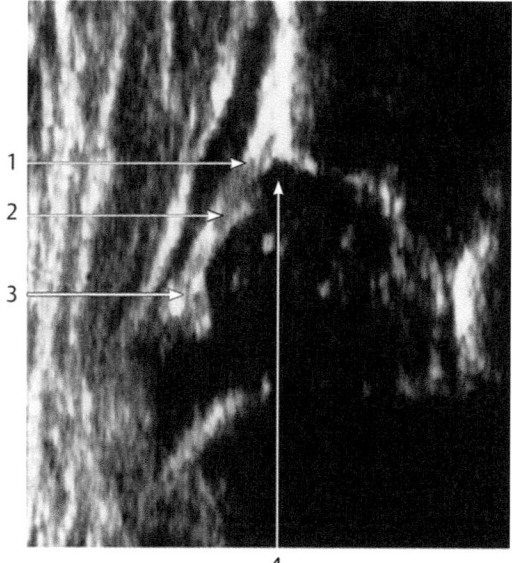

Fig. 3.22 Synovial fold. The synovial fold appears as two parallel echo stripes (1 = perichondrium, 2 = labrum, 3 = synovial fold, 4 = cartilaginous acetabular roof)

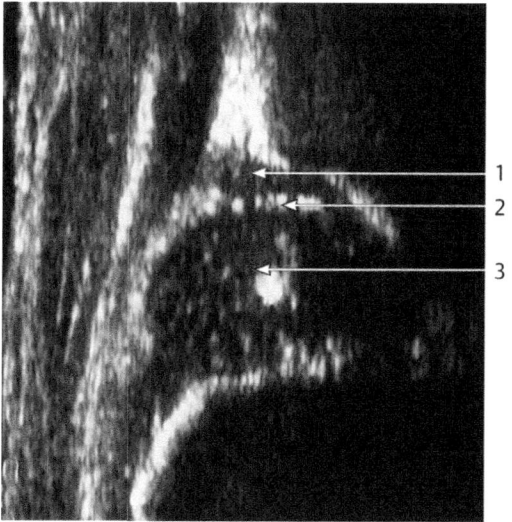

Fig. 3.23 Vacuum phenomenon. Hip sonogram of a 6-month-old child. The vacuum phenomenon (previously mistakenly called the fluid film) clearly delineates the femoral head against the hyaline cartilage of the acetabular roof (1 = hyaline cartilage of the acetabular roof, 2 = vacuum phenomenon, 3 = femoral head)

the echo of the labrum can be found lying inside the joint capsule, next to the hypoechoic structure of the hyaline cartilage of the acetabular roof, and further medially followed by the strong echo of the bony acetabulum and the structures of the acetabular fossa.

Vacuum Phenomenon ("Fluid Film")
In most cases, the femoral head is so close to the cartilaginous acetabular roof that the narrow joint space cannot be seen sonographically. However, on some sonograms a delicate, curved echo stripe can be seen at the boundary between the femoral head and the hyaline cartilaginous acetabular roof (see Fig. 3.23). These echoes are called the vacuum phenomenon, and created by nitrogen gas bubbles, which were formerly erroneously referred to as a fluid film (see Fig. 3.24).

If the vacuum phenomenon is seen sonographically, the hyaline cartilage of the femoral head can be separated from the hyaline cartilage of the acetabulum, so that the entire upper circumference of the femoral head is visible.

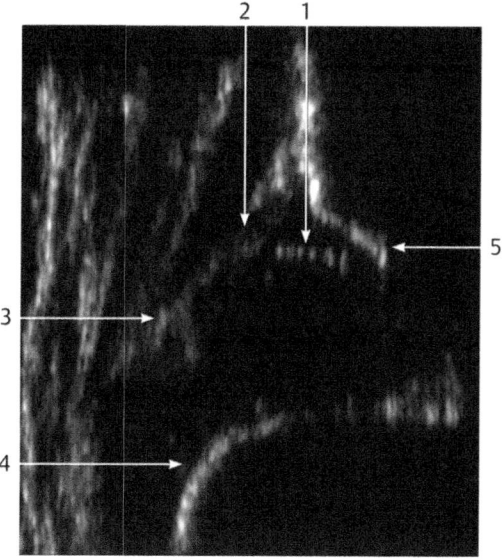

Fig. 3.24 Vacuum phenomenon newborn hip (1 = vacuum phenomenon, 2 = perichondrial gap with underlying labrum, 3 = synovial fold, 4 = chondro-osseous border, 5 = lower limb of the ilium bone)

Possibilities for Error
Caution

Often, the echo of the synovial fold is confused with the echo of the labrum.

If one follows the joint capsule starting from the synovial fold, it is important to ensure that one does not mistakenly follow the echo of an intermuscular septum instead of the joint capsule. Unfortunately, this confusion is not infrequently encountered in Type-III or Type-IV joints.

3.3.5 Summary

Conclusion

- Chondro-osseous border:
  - Arcuate.
  - with sound palisades.
  - only lateral part (medial not visible).
- Femoral head:
  - not round.
  - sinusoids.
  - zona anularis.
  - zona centralis.
- Ossific nucleus:
  - not round.
  - not in the centre of the head, visible on ultrasound before visible on X-ray.
  - Problems:
    - half-moon sign.
    - limits the technique.
    - size determination not possible.

3.4 Acetabular Fossa and Acetabular Roof

3.4.1 Acetabular Fossa

The floor of the acetabulum, the acetabular fossa (see Fig. 3.25), is formed by three bones:

- the lower part of the os ilium.
- the os ischium.
- the os pubis.

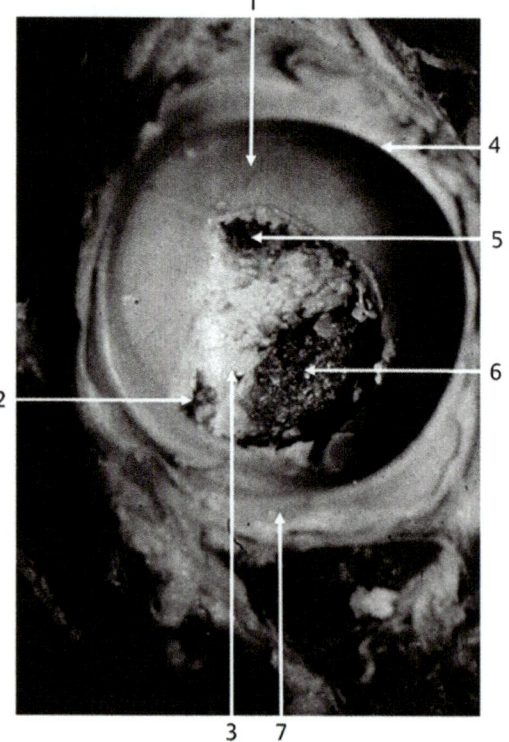

Fig. 3.25 Top view of the left acetabulum. Specimen from a 3-month-old infant. The ligamentum teres and the tissue of the acetabular fossa have been excised, exposing the acetabular floor (1 = lunate surface of the acetabulum, 2 = pubic bone, 3 = descending branch of triradiate cartilage, 4 = labrum, 5 = ilium, 6 = ischium, 7 = acetabular notch with the transverse ligament)

The three bones, forming the acetabular fossa are connected by the hyaline cartilaginous Y-shaped triradiate growth plate. The acetabular fossa is lined with fat and connective tissue. Between this tissue and the femoral head, the ligamentum teres stretches from the region of the acetabular notch (incisura acetabuli) upwards. It attaches with a relatively broad insertion at the fovea centralis of the femoral head (see Fig. 3.26a). Located within the ligamentum teres is the artery that enters under the transverse acetabular ligament into the teres ligament and thus arises outside the joint space. With high-resolution ultrasound machines, it is possible to display the blood flow and the pulse wave in the artery of the teres ligament (see Fig. 3.26b) [11].

The transverse acetabular ligament is located lateral to the ligamentum teres and is the extension of the three dimensional structure of the labrum over the acetabular notch (see Fig. 3.27).

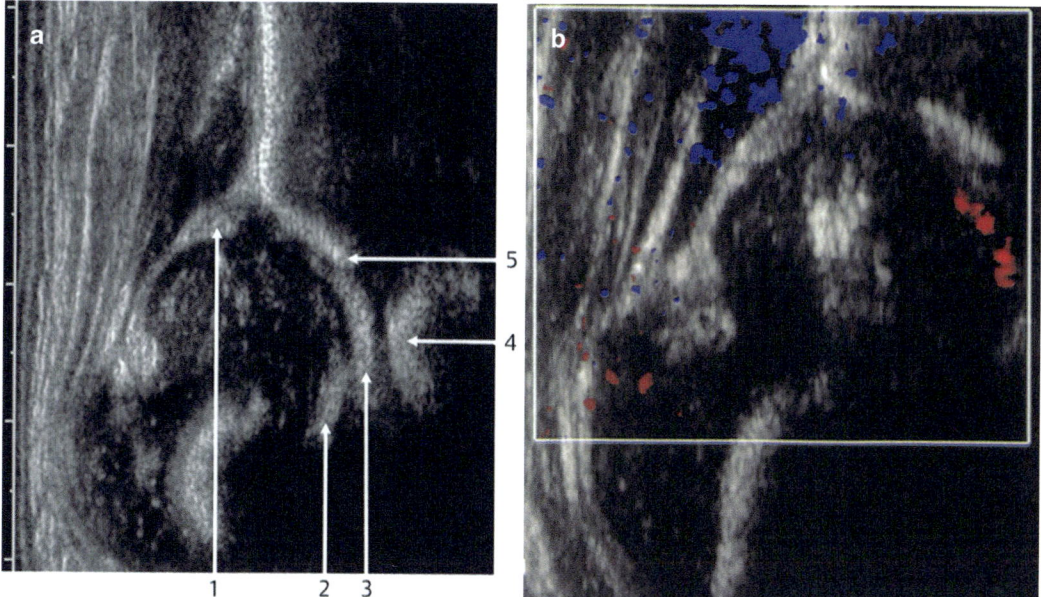

Fig. 3.26 Ligamentum teres (1 = labrum, 2 = transverse ligament, 3 = ligamentum teres, 4 = ischium, 5 = lower limb of the os ilium, (**a**) The teres ligament is clearly vis- ible in the sonogram (**b**) The artery within the teres liga- ment can be clearly visualized in the colour Doppler sonogram)

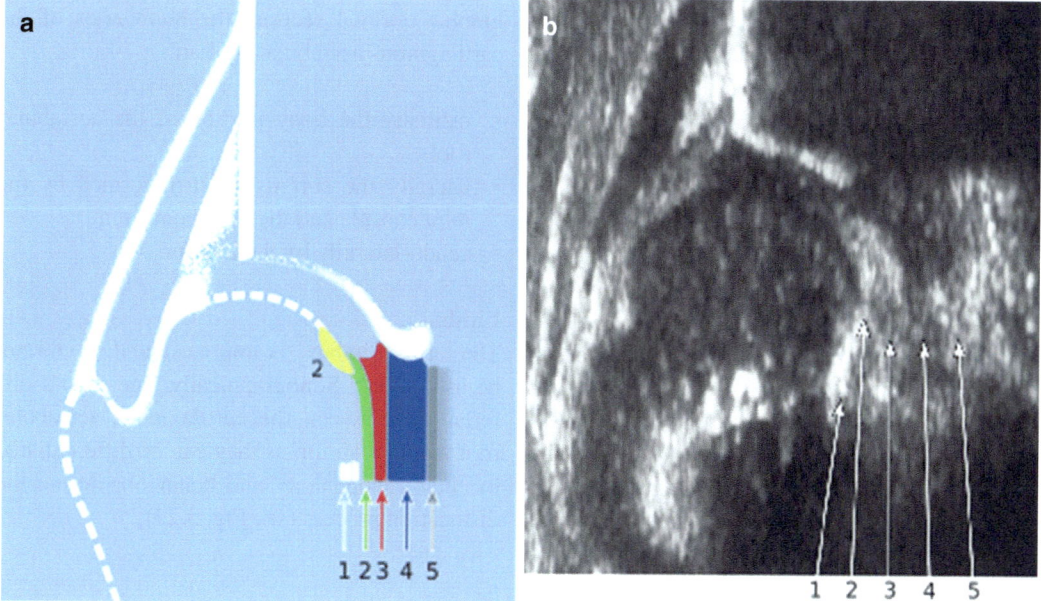

Fig. 3.27 1 = transverse ligament, 2 = ligamentum teres and central fovea, 3 = fat tissue of the acetabular fossa, 4 = triradiate cartilage (growth plate), 5 = perichondrium on the inner side of the pelvis, (**a**) Schematic representa- tion of the ligament, (**b**) Sonogram of a newborn with a good view into the acetabular fossa

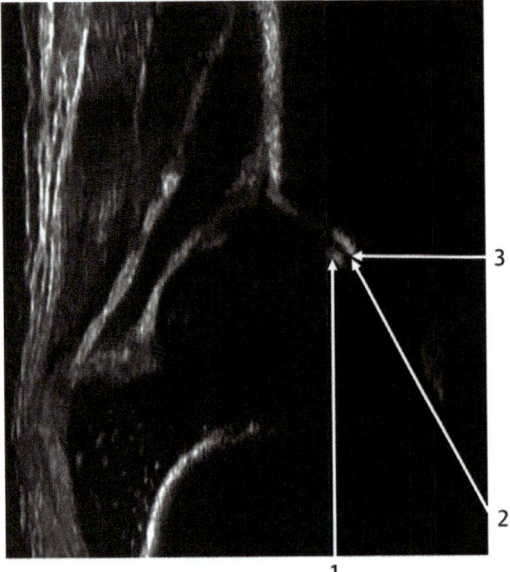

Fig. 3.28 Typical three-layered echo in the depth of the acetabular fossa (1 = ligamentum teres with fovea centralis, 2 = weak echoes of the fatty tissue of the acetabular fossa (hypoechoic zone), 3 = lower limb of the iliac bone)

Sonographically, the lower limb of the os ilium appears as a strong, reflective echo, and caudal to the lower limb is the hypoechoic zone of the triradiate cartilage. Lateral to that, usually appearing hypoechoic or nearly anechoic, depending on the fat content, is a zone of fat and connective tissue filling the acetabular fossa (pulvinar). The ligamentum teres appears as a bright echo, radiating into the fovea centralis, usually showing strong echogenicity.

A common error of mis-identification is a mix up between the lower limb of the os ilium and the fovea centralis. Both structures are usually equally echogenic, and it is not uncommon for the echo of the fovea centralis to be mis-identified as the lower limb of the os ilium. The structures can be separated as described above by dynamic examination, i.e. moving the hip, or by identifying their typical three-layer echogenicity (see Fig. 3.28):

- laterally, the fovea centralis.
- medially, the echo of the lower limb of the os ilium.
- between both structures, a hypoechoic zone, which corresponds to the fat and connective tissue.

3.4.2   Cartilaginous Acetabular Roof

Nomenclature

> Learning points: The hyaline cartilage acetabular roof is of central importance in hip ultrasonography.

All forms of disorders of hip maturation and dislocation leave their traces on the acetabular roof. Classification and typing are only possible if the structures on the bony, and especially on the cartilaginous acetabular roof, can be clearly and unambiguously identified even in markedly pathological cases. Unfortunately, the nomenclature is not uniform, particularly in the area of the acetabular roof.

The cartilaginous acetabular roof attaches to the bony acetabulum. The peripheral boundary of the cartilaginous acetabular roof is the fibrocartilaginous ring of the labrum. This projects freely into the joint and is only fused at its narrow base with the cartilaginous acetabular roof. In a sonographic coronal section, the boundaries of the cartilaginous acetabular roof are:

- medially the bony portion of the acetabular roof.
- laterally the soft tissue strip formed by the joint capsule and the perichondrium.
- caudo-laterally by the labrum.

Limbus
The term "Limbus" is imprecise and should not be used today. Sonographically, one should differentiate between the cartilaginous acetabular roof and the labrum as they can be differentiated by their echogenicity and behaviour during the dislocation process (see Fig. 3.29).

3.4.3   Boundaries and Special Sonographic Structure of the Hyaline Cartilage Roof

Anatomy
The cartilaginous roof is covered laterally by the perichondrium (see Fig. 3.30 and Fig. 3.31). The

Fig. 3.29 Structure of the acetabular roof

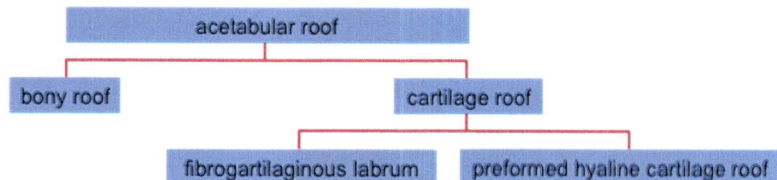

Fig. 3.30 Anatomy of the proximal perichondrium. Schematic representation (1 = perichondrium of the hyaline cartilage of the acetabular roof, 2 = labrum, 3 = joint capsule with ischiofemoral ligament, 4 = joint capsule next to the fat pad, 5 = tendon of the m. rectus femoris, reflected head)

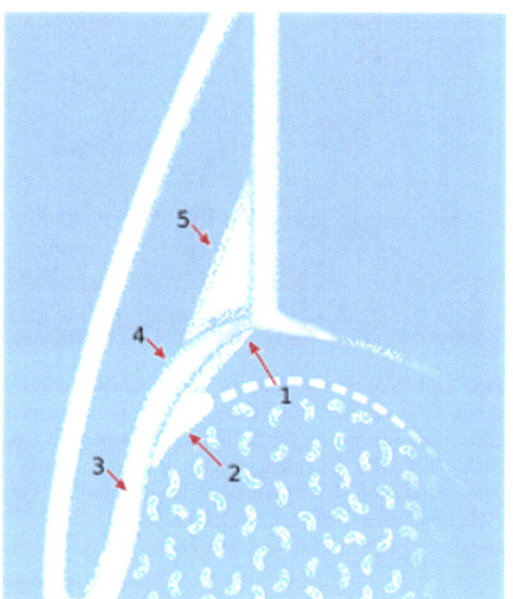

Fig. 3.31 Anatomy of the proximal perichondrium. Cadaveric specimen (1 = perichondrium of the hyaline cartilage of the acetabular roof, 2 = labrum, 3 = joint capsule with ischiofemoral ligament, 4 = joint capsule next to the fat pad, 5 = tendon of the reflected head of the rectus femoris muscle)

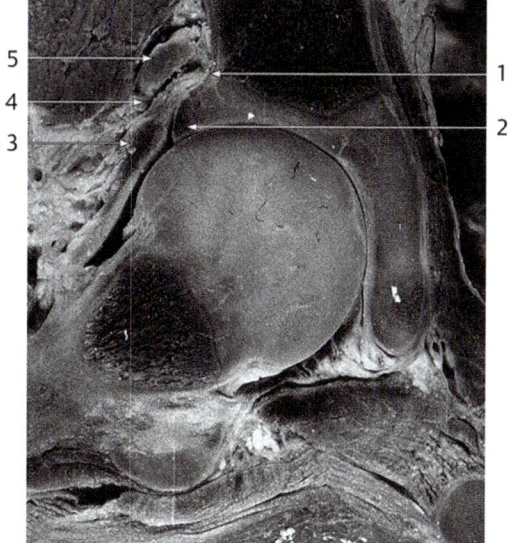

next structure lateral to that is the joint capsule extending cranially from the synovial fold, ending in the fat pad, which can be recognized in the sonogram as a hypoechoic strip. Lateral to this hypoechoic strip, which is the fat pad of the joint capsule, there is a strong echo in the upper portion of the cartilage roof: this is the reflected head of the rectus femoris muscle.

Within the joint capsule itself, at the level of the labrum, there is often an area of increased echogenicity. This is the ischiofemoral ligament (see Fig. 3.32). This structure must not be confused with the labrum or even misinterpreted as a "ruptured labrum."

Sonographic Identification

With high-resolution machines, the three anatomical structures described above can be identified separately, which, due to their close proximity (see Fig. 3.33), often appear as one summation echo and are referred to as the proximal perichondrium (see Fig. 3.34). The labrum continues to be visible as a strong echo on the inside of the joint capsule and is sometimes separated from the joint capsule by a recess, which can be seen sonographically. Proximal to the echo of the labrum and the ischiofemoral ligament on the one hand and distal to the strong echo of the so-called proximal perichondrium on the other, there is reduced echo-

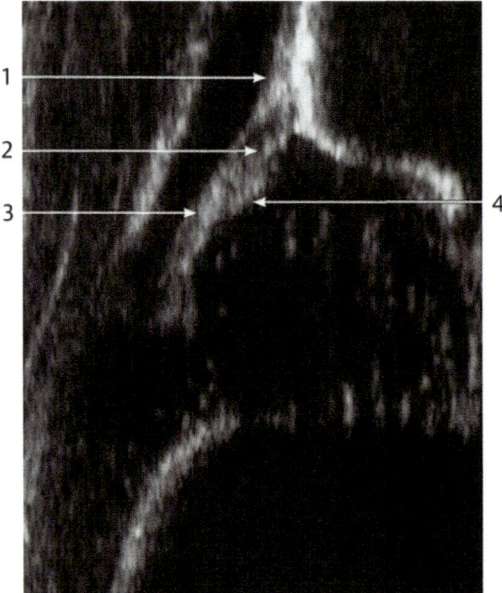

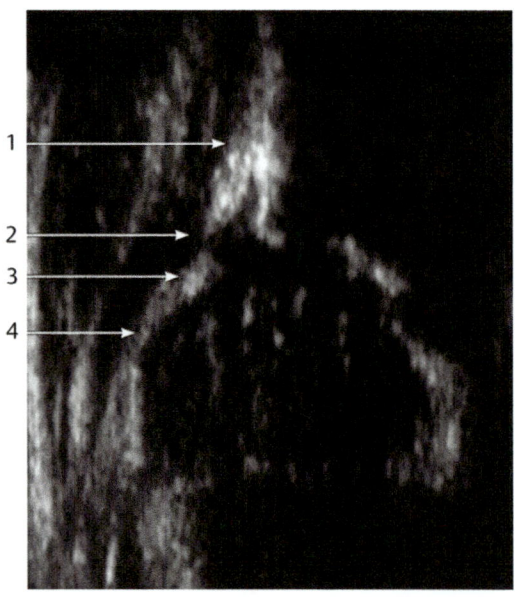

Fig. 3.32 Sonographic identification of the proximal perichondrium (1 = rectus tendon, 2 = joint capsule attachment with fat pad and perichondrium, 3 = ischiofemoral ligament, 4 = labrum)

Fig. 3.34 Summation echo of the proximal perichondrium. The structures in the area of the proximal perichondrium can no longer be accurately separated from each other. The proximal perichondrium appears as a summation echo (1 = proximal perichondrium, 2 = perichondrial gap, 3 = labrum, 4 = joint capsule)

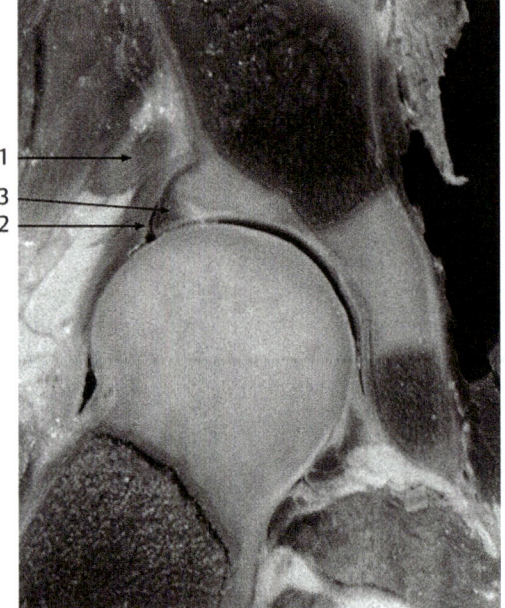

Fig. 3.33 Oblique section through the area of the acetabular roof. The separation between the rectus femoris muscle and the joint capsule with the ischiofemoral ligament is not clearly seen (1 = rectus femoris muscle, 2 = ischiofemoral ligament, 3 = labrum).

genicity, so this area is referred to as the "perichondrial gap" (see Fig. 3.35 and Fig. 3.34).

The relative reduction in echogenicity that led to the term perichondrial gap [12] is due to the weak echoes of the distal part of the perichondrium and the thin joint capsule on the one hand, and the strong echo of the attachment of the rectus tendon (caput reflexum) on the other hand.

> **Learning point**
>
> - Proximal perichondrium: The proximal perichondrium is a summation echo. and consists of the perichondrium of the cartilaginous acetabular roof, the joint capsule, and the attachment of the reflexed head of the rectus femoris muscle. (see Fig. 3.36).
> - Perichondrial gap: The so-called perichondrial gap arises due to the poor reflectivity compared to the echo of the rectus tendon and the echo of the ischiofemoral ligament.

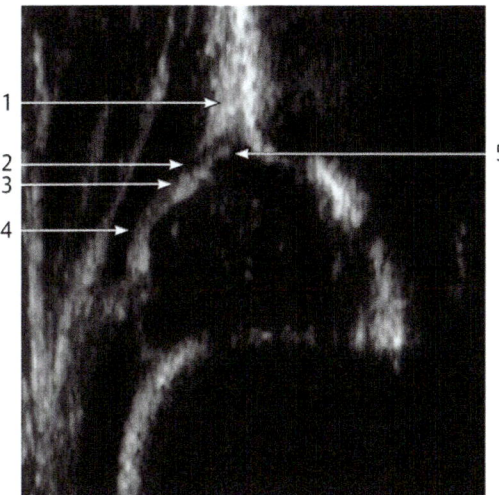

Fig. 3.35 Separation of the proximal perichondrium (1 = origin of rectus tendon, 2 = perichondrial gap, 3 = labrum, 4 = joint capsule, 5 = perichondrium of the hyaline cartilage of the acetabular roof)

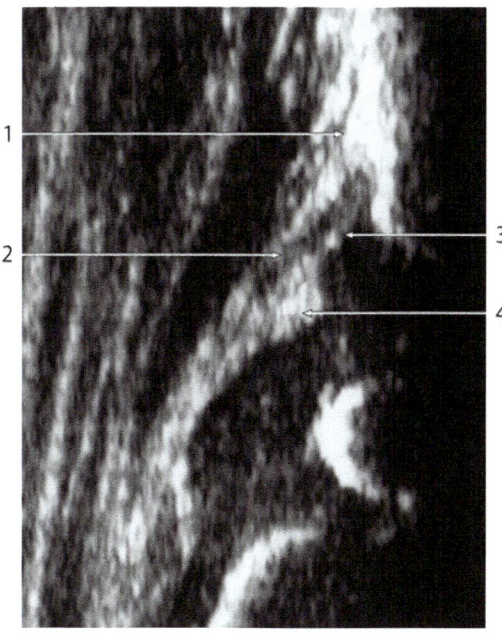

Fig. 3.36 Proximal perichondrium (1 = attachment of the rectus tendon, 2 = joint capsule next to the hypoechoic zone of the fat pad, 3 = perichondrium of the hyaline cartilage of the acetabular roof, 4 = labrum)

3.4.4 Summary

Conclusion

- Acetabular fossa:
  - three bones.
  - Y-shaped growth plate (triradiate cartilage).
  - covered with connective tissue.
  - ligamentum teres.
  - transverse ligament (bridges the acetabular notch).
- Perichondrium:
  - Proximal perichondrium:
    - perichondrium.
    - joint capsule (fat pad of the joint capsule).
    - reflected head of the rectus femoris muscle (Caput reflexum).
  - Perichondrial gap: Caudal area of the perichondrium with weaker, less reflective echoes.

3.5 Pathology of the Acetabulum

Except in cases of teratological hip dislocation, the decentering femoral head causes specific changes in the bone during the dislocation process, but even more so in the cartilaginous roof of the acetabulum. In other words, when the femoral head dislocates from the acetabulum, it leaves very characteristic "abrasion marks" on the socket—both on the cartilaginous and the bony part. If it is now possible to classify the different stages of the abrasion marks on the acetabulum by type, then these types represent a snapshot of the dynamic dislocation process.

3.5.1 Morphological Changes During the Dislocation Process

For a better understanding of the sonographic images in hip maturation disorders, the anatomical and histological findings during the dislocation process have been described. Detailed morphological studies were published by Bernbeck [13], Oelkers [14, 15], Dörr [16], and Ponseti [17]. Further changes in the early embryonic pelvis with the loss of the guiding function of the acetabulum were extensively described in the literature [9, 15, 17]. The histomorphological changes during the dislocation process were also documented in detail [14, 15].

During the dislocation process caused by caudo-cranial shear forces [18–21], the base of the labrum forms a stable fulcrum (Hypomochlion) [14, 15], while the tip of the labrum is pushed upwards (see Fig. 3.37 and Fig. 3.38).

Evidence of a fibrocartilaginous labrum that is folded inwards can only be found in the rare case of a teratological dislocation that occurred in the early foetal period, [17]. Dörr also came to the same conclusion during his macroscopic examinations of the DDH specimens from the Ortolani collection [16].

> **Learning point**
>
> It is important to recognize that the base of the labrum is secured to the cartilage roof by circumferential fibres (see Fig. 3.39 and see Fig. 3.40). These fibres provide special stability to this region.

3.5.2 Histological Changes at the Acetabulum

At the transition zone between the hyaline cartilage acetabular roof and the bony acetabulum, there is a growth area. This area is characterized by the regular columnar cartilage structure that is typical of a chondro-osseous border or growth plate (see Fig. 3.41).

In decentred hip joints, pressure and shearing forces induce pathomorphological changes at the

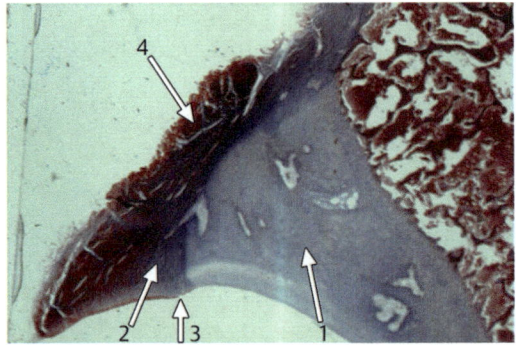

Fig. 3.37 Hip dislocation (**a**) Hip joint with secondary socket and original acetabulum (1 = secondary socket, 2 = original acetabulum, 3 = so-called Neolimbus according to Ortolani), (**b**) Histological sect. (1 = base of labrum compressed downwards, 2 = cranio-dorsally deformed labrum, 3 = hyaline cartilage roof), (**c**) X-ray image. (1 = part of the cartilage roof compressed downwards, 2 = tip of the cranially flattened labrum, 3 = original acetabulum)

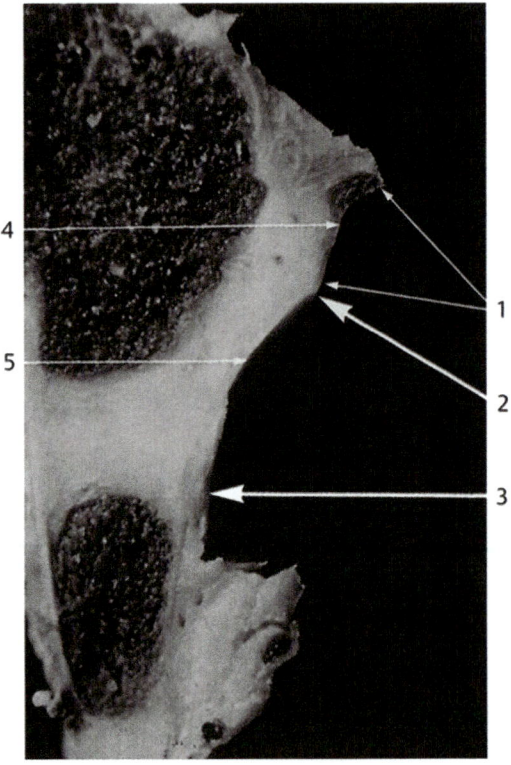

Fig. 3.38 Reduced femoral head in various positions (1 = acetabular cartilage 2 = components of the cartilage roof) (**a**) Incomplete reduction: the femoral head is pressed against the acetabular cartilage which is pushed downwards. (**b**) Ideal reposition through flexion and moderate abduction (**c**) The components of the roof with the acetabular cartilage partially pressed downwards and the cartilage roof elongated upwards are clearly visible

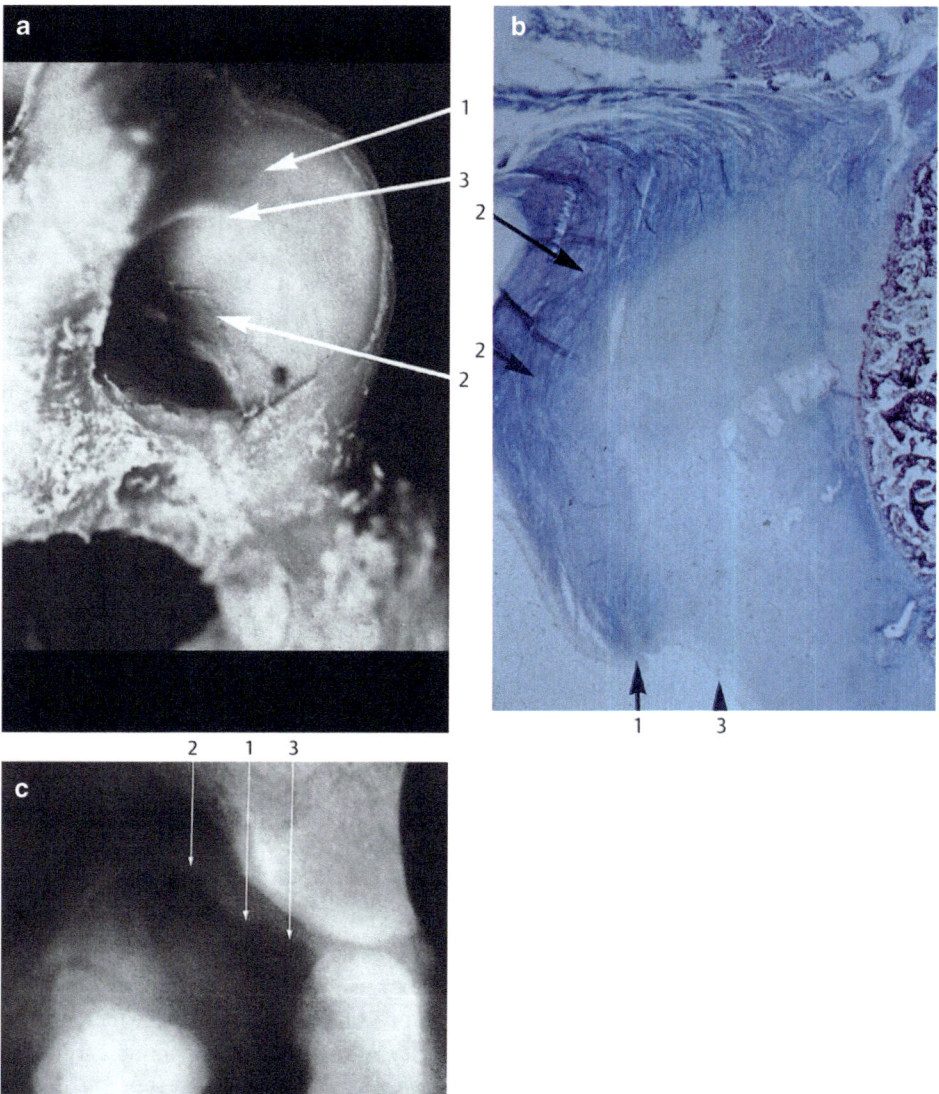

Fig. 3.39 Section through the cartilaginous portion of the acetabular roof. The hyaline cartilage of the acetabular roof is next to the bony socket. The labrum is particularly firmly fixed at its base to the cartilage of the acetabular roof with collagen fibres (1 = hyaline cartilage of the acetabular roof, 2 = labrum, 3 = base of the labrum, 4 = joint capsule)

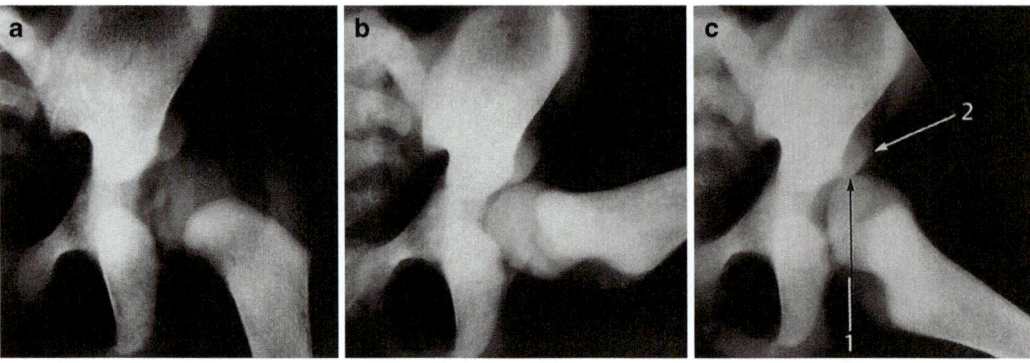

Fig. 3.40 Macroscopic section through a dislocated hip. The labrum, displaced upwards, and the fulcrum point (base of the labrum) are clearly visible (1 = labrum, 2 = base of the labrum, 3 = acetabular fossa, 4 = secondary socket with flattened labrum, 5 = facies lunata (so-called original socket)

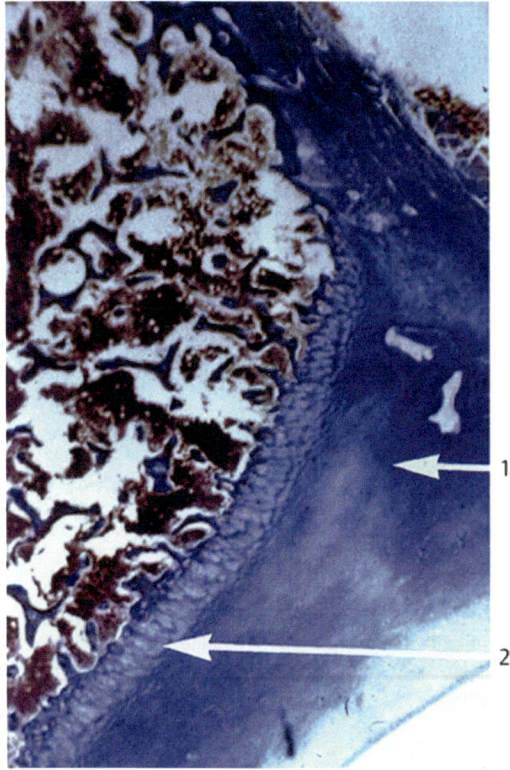

Fig. 3.41 Histology of the region of the acetabular roof in a healthy hip joint. The hyaline cartilage of the acetabular roof is separated from the bony acetabular roof by a columnar cartilage growth zone (1 = hyaline cartilage of the acetabular roof, 2 = growth zone)

growth plate of the acetabular roof that lead to growth arrest and progressive flattening of the bony acetabulum (see Fig. 3.42) [22]. These caudo-cranial shearing forces, caused by the dislocating femoral head, deform the non-ossified cartilaginous roof in a typical way [23].

With further deformation of the relatively soft cartilaginous acetabular roof, dislocation of the femoral head inevitably occurs. Klisic coined the term "Developmental Dysplasia of the Hip" [24], which describes this development, replacing the term "Congenital Dislocation of the Hip."

Moreover, under the influence of pressure, histological transformation of chondrocytes into fibrocytes can occur in the cartilage roof. In regions of increased pressure, the normal histological structure of the hyaline cartilage of the acetabular roof can be lost (see Fig. 3.43). Once this histological transformation or degeneration reaches a certain extent, it can, at least in part, also be detected sonographically (see Type IIIb). The most important consequence of these findings must be the indication for early treatment.

Beware

Diagnosis and, if necessary, treatment should be started as early as possible before pressure and shearing forces irreversibly destroy the histology of the acetabular cartilage and the growth plate.

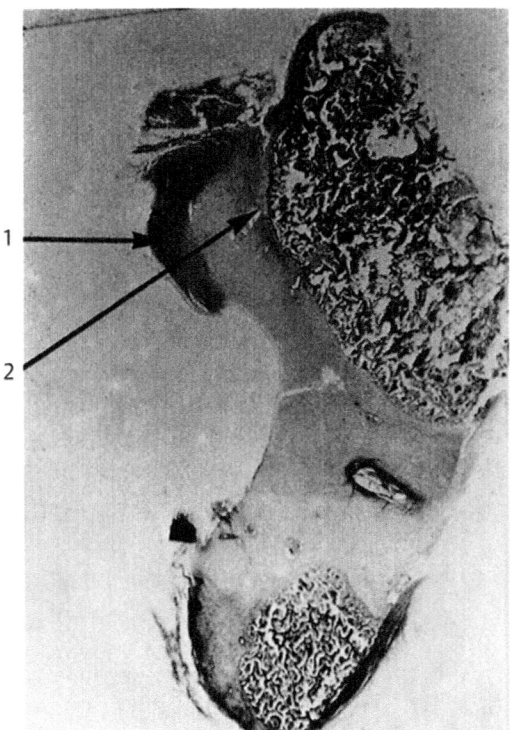

Fig. 3.42 Cross-section of the right acetabulum. The acetabular labrum is displaced upwards by the joint capsule and the cartilaginous acetabular roof is deformed. The regular columnar cartilage of the growth zone has been largely destroyed by compressive and shearing forces (for comparison, see Fig. 3.41). (1 = labrum, 2 = growth area)

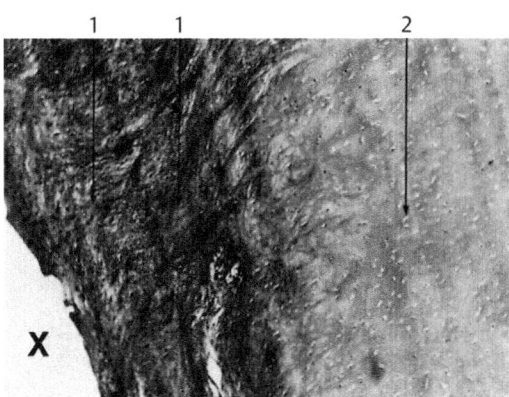

Fig. 3.43 Acetabular roof cartilage with a decentred femoral head. Significant remodelling due to unmasking of the collagen fibres. The position of the dislocated femoral head is marked with an "X". The acetabular roof cartilage outside the compression zone has not yet undergone histological changes (1 = cartilaginous portion with damaged structure (compression zone) 2 = histologically unremarkable cartilage)

References

1. Anderhuber F. Embryologie und Morphogenese. In: Tschauner C, editor. Die Hüfte. Stuttgart: Enke; 1997. p. 1–3.
2. Graf R. Sonographie der Säuglingshüfte und therapeutische Konsequenzen. 6th ed. Stuttgart: Thieme; 2010.
3. Suzuki S, Kasahara Y, Futami T, et al. Ultrasonography in congenital dislocation of the hip: simultaneous imaging of both hips from in front. J Bone Joint Surg Br. 1991;73-B:879–83.
4. Graf R, Tschauner C. Ultrasound screening in the neonatal period. Baillièrés Clin Orthop. 1996;1(1):117–33.
5. Dorn U, Hattwich M. Die sonographische Beurteilung der Schenkelhalsantetorsion. Orthop Praxis. 1986;22:248–53.
6. Putti V. Early treatment of congenital dislocation of the hip. J Bone Joint Surg. 1929;17:798–812.
7. Hilgenreiner WH. Zur Frühdiagnose und Frühbehandlung der angeborenen Hüftgelenksverrenkung. Med Klin. 1925;21(1385–1389):1425–9.
8. Tönnis D. Die angeborene Hüftdysplasie und Hüftluxation im Kindes- und Erwachsenenalter. Berlin: Springer; 1984.
9. Batory I. Ätiologie der pathologischen Veränderungen des kindlichen Hüftgelenkes. Stuttgart: Enke; 1982.
10. Harcke HT, Clarke NMP, Lee MS, et al. Examination of the infant hip with real-time ultrasonography. J Ultrasound Med. 1984;3:131–7.
11. Graf R, Lercher K. Erfahrungen mit einem 3-D-Sonographiesystem am Säuglingshüftgelenk. Ultraschall Med. 1996;17:218–24.
12. Graf R. The ultrasonic image of the acetabular rim in infants. An experimental and clinical investigation. Arch Orthop Traumat. 1981;99:35–41.
13. Bernbeck R. Zur Pathologie der Luxatio coxae congenita. Virchow Arch Pathol Anat. 1951;320:238–52.
14. Oelkers H. Die Sauerstofffüllung zur Diagnostik und Indikationsstellung bei der angeborenen Hüftluxation. Verh Dtsch Orthop Ges 48. Kongreß Z Orthop 1961; 94: 327.
15. Oelkers H. Histologischer und röntgenologischer Vergleich zwischen einem dysplastischen Becken (Luxationsbecken) und Normalbefund. Orthop Praxis. 1981;17:614–24.
16. Dörr WM. Makroskopisch-anatomische, osteologische und röntgenologische Untersuchungen an frühkindlichen Hüft- luxationspräparaten [Habilitationsschrift]. Aachen: Univer- sität Aachen; 1968.
17. Ponseti IV. Growth and development of the acetabulum in the normal child and morphology of the acetabulum in congenital dislocation of the hip. J Bone Joint Surg. 1978;60-A:575–99.
18. Matthiessen HD. Die „endogene" Hüftdysplasie. In: Schilt M, Hrsg. Angeborene Hüftdysplasie und -luxation vom Neugeborenen bis zum Erwachsenen. Zürich: SGUMB- SVUPP-Eigenverlag; 1993a: 117–133.

19. Matthiessen HD. Dynamik des Wachstums im Pfannen- dach. In: Schilt M, editor. Angeborene Hüftdysplasie und -lu- xation vom Neugeborenen bis zum Erwachsenen. Zürich: SGUMB-SVUPP-Eigenverlag; 1993b. p. 19–46.
20. Matthiessen HD. Forensische Probleme bei der Behandlung von Hüftdysplasien und -luxationen. Z Orthop. 1996;134:10–2.
21. Matthiessen HD. Dysplasie- und Therapiefaktor bei der Hüftreifungsstörung. Z Orthop. 1997;135:12–3.
22. Graf R, Hammer N, Matthiesen D. An integrated concept explaining for risk factors related to the onset of developmental dysplasia of the hip joint. Ann Orthop Musculo- skelet Disord. 2021;4(1):1029.
23. Rodegerts U, Matthiessen HD. Wachstumskinetik und His- tomorphometrik der Wachstumsfuge. II. Symposium des SFB 1988. Teratologische Forschung und Rehabilitation mehrfach Behinderter der WWU Münster 1971; 2: 551–556.
24. Klisic P. Let's adopt the term: "Developmental displacement of the hip" (DDH). Proceedings No 86 of international meeting on care of babies' hips. Beograd 01.–03.10.1987.

Step-by-Step Approach to Hip Sonography

4

4.1 Anatomical Identification (Checklist I)

In every evaluation of a hip sonogram, the identification of the anatomical structures is crucial. A precise step-by-step approach can prevent confusion and incorrect identification of important anatomical structures—54% of incorrect diagnoses are based on incorrect anatomical identification.

4.1.1 Chondro-Osseous Border, Femoral Head, Synovial Fold, and Joint Capsule

The identification begins with the following steps:

1. Step 1: First, locate the chondro-osseous border. Following the chondro-osseous border medially, one arrives at the hypoechoic femoral head.
2. Step 2: After identifying the femoral head, the echo of the synovial fold is located lateral to the femoral head and proximal to the chondro-osseous border.
3. Step 3: After identifying the synovial fold, follow the joint capsule proximally to the labrum.
4. Step 4: Once the labrum has been identified, it must be verified as the actual echo of the labrum, using the labrum definitions.

> **Learning point:**
> To step 3: In pathological cases, the intermuscular septum is often mistaken for the joint capsule.

4.1.2 The Labrum

The intraarticular structure of the labrum projects into the joint with a triangular shape that touches but is not fused with the inner side of the joint capsule (see Fig. 4.1). There is a small fatty recess between the joint capsule and the labrum (see Fig. 4.2).

The labrum is only attached to the hyaline cartilage roof of the acetabulum. Sonographically, it can sometimes be difficult to identify the position of the labrum. However, in order to locate it correctly even in difficult situations, the four labrum definitions [1, 2] can be used to help with the identification process, but they do not have to be applied at the same time. A single labrum definition is enough to identify the labrum with certainty.

Definitions for the Labrum

- The labrum is always in contact with the femoral head.
- The labrum is the most lateral part of the hyaline cartilage roof, inside the joint capsule.

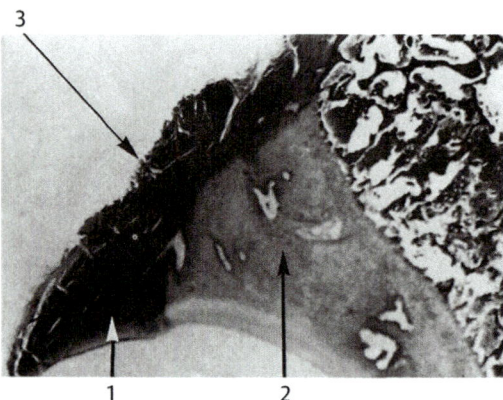

Fig. 4.1 Histological cross-section through the cartilaginous and bony acetabulum of a right hip (1 = labrum, 2 = hyaline cartilage roof, 3 = joint capsule and perichondrium)

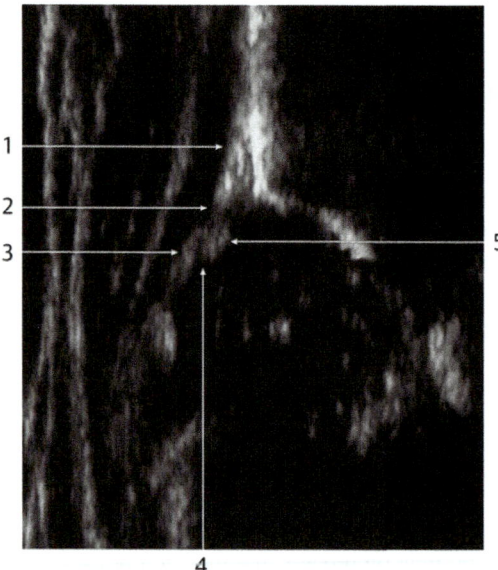

Fig. 4.2 Sonogram with clearly visible perilabral recess (1 = proximal perichondrium, 2 = perichondrial gap, 3 = joint capsule, 4 = perilabral recess, 5 = labrum)

- The labrum is located caudal to the perichondrial gap.
- The labrum is in the corner, where the joint capsule diverges from the surface of the femoral head.

4.1.3   Standard Sequence

After identifying the chondro-osseous border, the femoral head, the synovial fold, the joint capsule, and the labrum, the standard sequence follows:

If one follows the surface of the femoral head from lateral to medial after identifying the labrum, the next structure after the labrum is the hyaline cartilage roof. Further medial, the echoes of the bony socket can be identified.

Order from lateral to medial:

- labrum
- cartilage roof
- bony roof (not bony rim)

The order of Labrum–Cartilage–Bone is called the standard sequence (refer to Fig. 4.3). The order of structures remains essentially unchanged, even in pathological hip joints.

Therefore, the standard sequence should always be applied: the reference points should be identified in the following order (Fig. 4.4):

- chondro-osseous border
- femoral head
- synovial fold
- joint capsule
- labrum
- cartilage (hyaline cartilage)
- bony roof

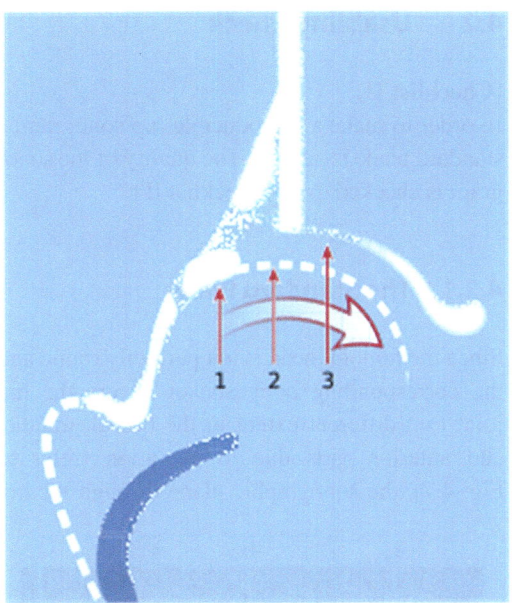

Fig. 4.3 Standard sequence. The standard sequence refers to the order Labrum–Cartilage–Bone (1 = labrum, 2 = cartilage, 3 = bone)

4.1.4   Turning Point

The turning point is the most lateral point of the bony roof's concavity. By definition, it is the point at which the bony roof of the acetabulum transitions from the concavity of the acetabulum to the convexity of the ilium (see Fig. 4.5).

> **Learning point**
> Short definition: The turning point is the transition point where the concavity turns to convexity.

It is important always to start with the concavity, meaning to search for the turning point from distal-medial to proximal-lateral (from bottom to top). Additionally, an acoustic shadow can often be observed at the turning point (Fig. 4.6). The turning point is the most lateral point of the acoustic shadow.

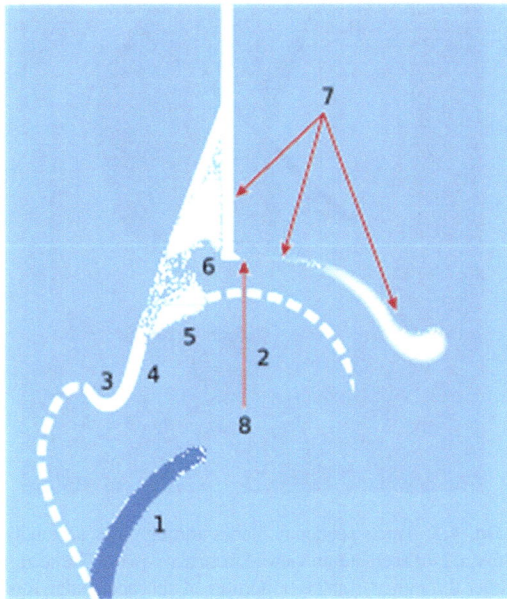

Fig. 4.4 Anatomical identification (Checklist I). The anatomical structures must be identified in the correct order (1 chondro-osseous border, 2 femoral head, 3 synovial fold, 4 joint capsule, 5 labrum, 6 cartilage (cartilaginous roof), 7 bone (bony roof), 8 concavity to convexity (determination of the turning point). The concavity of the acetabulum turns into the convexity of the ilium. Brief definition: Concavity–Convexity

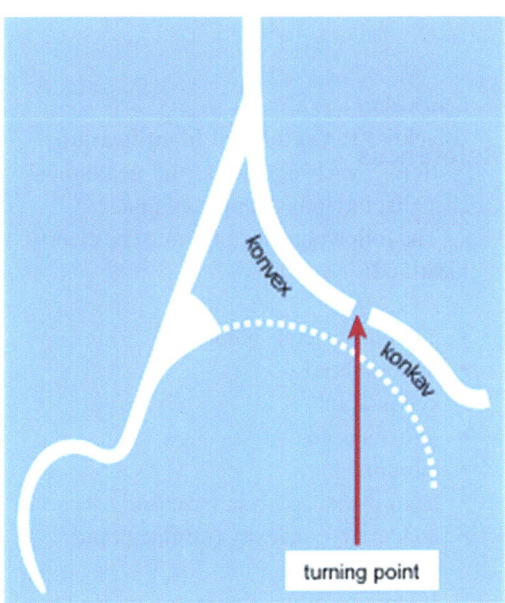

Fig. 4.5 Identification of the turning point. Schematic picture showing the turning point, where the acetabular concavity turns to convexity

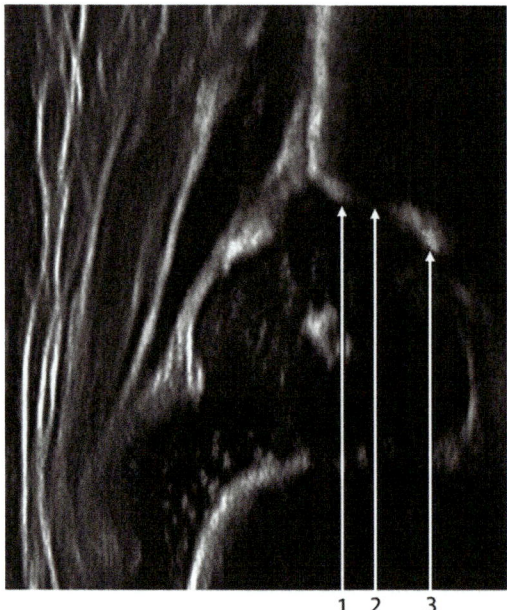

Fig. 4.6 Identification of the turning point. Transition from concavity to convexity. The turning point is the most lateral point of the acoustic shadow (1 = turning point, 2 = acoustic shadow, 3 = lower limb of the ilium)

4.1.5 Checklist I

Conclusion
Checklist I: Anatomical Identification.

   Before each diagnosis, the anatomical checklist has to be completed first.

   The following structures must be clearly identified:

- chondro-osseous border
- femoral head
- synovial fold
- joint capsule
- labrum
- labrum–cartilage–bone (standard sequence)
- concavity–convexity (turning point)

   If any one of the above structures is not identified, the sonogram should not be used for diagnosis.

4.2   Usability Check

(Checklist II)
In order to make a reproducible hip sonogram, a standard plane is needed. The quality of the sonogram is checked using Checklist II.

4.2.1   The Standard Plane

Since the femoral head is not perfectly round and the corresponding bony socket covers the hip joint to a different extent in the dorsal, middle, and anterior parts due to evolution (refer to Fig. 4.7), the sonographic plane through the hip

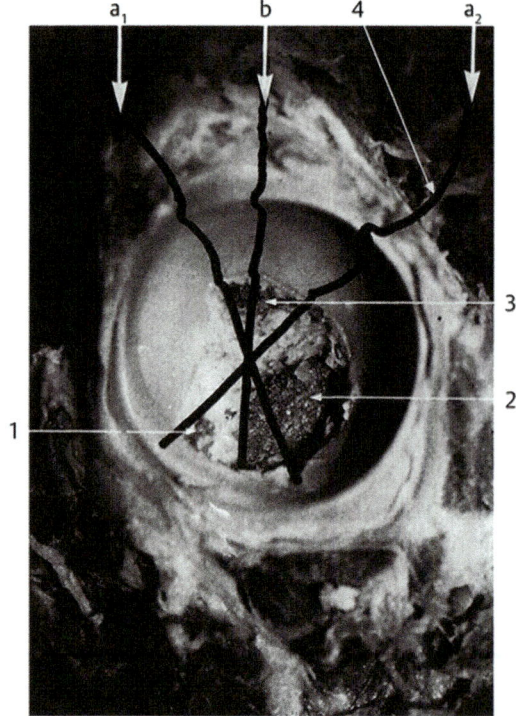

Fig. 4.7 Three sectional planes through the acetabular fossa. Left acetabulum viewed from above a1 = The section cuts through the anterior portion of the acetabular roof, a2 = The section cuts through the posterior portion of the acetabular roof and into the concavity of the gluteal fossa, b = correct mid plane. 1 = Os pubis, 2 = Os ischium, 3 = Os ilium, 4 = Concavity of the gluteal fossa. "No success in hip sonography without the lower limb"—there is only one exception to this rule: in the case of decentred joints, sometimes the lower limb of the ilium is not visible on the sonogram. The femoral head dislocates dorso-cranially and is located outside of the standard plane (see Fig. 4.13a).

joint must be precisely determined. Otherwise, reproducible cross-sections through the hip joint cannot be obtained.

A plane can be spatially defined with three points in a three-dimensional space.

In relation to a hip sonogram, the standard plane is defined by the following three landmarks:

- lower limb of the ilium
- middle portion of the acetabular roof corresponding to a coronal plane (later to be the weight-bearing zone)
- labrum

Landmark 1: Lower limb of the os ilium

Practical tip: In order for a description of the acetabulum to be meaningful, the sonographic standard plane has to go through the middle (weight-bearing) portion of the acetabular roof.

The lower limb is the part of the os ilium that lies in the acetabular fossa and is not covered by the lunate surface (see Fig. 4.7). Thus, sonographically, it forms the centre of the acetabulum. If the lower limb of the ilium is missing in the sonogram, this means, exaggeratedly, that the sonographic section was not even made through the hip joint. In this case, further assessment of the plane and the labrum is unnecessary as the position of these structures can only be correctly identified, if the lower limb of the ilium is visible, as it is the centre of the acetabulum, the pivot point for the sonographic plane. Therefore, when scanning, we must always look for the lower limb of the ilium before we look for the correct plane and labrum.

Landmark 2: Sectional plane through the acetabular roof.
If the lower limb of the ilium is visible, the first basic principle, that the sonographic plane is

through the middle of the acetabulum, is fulfilled.

Regarding the issue of the correct plane through the acetabular roof: ultrasound allows for an overview of the entire circumference of the roof resembling a tomogram.

During evolution, the pelvic rotation needed to transition from walking on four legs to an upright position, which means that the dorsal portions of the bony acetabulum are better developed than the middle and ventral portions. This means that depending on the choice of the sectional plane through the roof, completely different roof coverage, ranging from very good dorsally to poor bony coverage ventrally can be observed.

To be able to decide whether the sectional plane has intersected the anterior, middle, or posterior portion of the roof, the presence of the lower limb of the ilium through which the axis of rotation occurs, is essential (see Fig. 4.10). Once the lower limb is visualised, the typical appearances of the iliac bone can be assigned to the anterior, middle, and posterior part of the roof.

Characteristics of the Posterior Plane
The silhouette of the ilium proximal to the bony rim appears concave and inclines away from the ultrasound transducer in the upright projection. The concave shape corresponds to the gluteal fossa. Additionally, the area of the bony rim, corresponding to the dorsal crest of the acetabulum, is usually rounded in a "beak-like" shape (see Fig. 4.8a).

Characteristics of the Middle Plane
The silhouette of the ilium is a straight line and, assuming a standardized positioning device (cradle) and scanning technique (ultrasound probe guide) are used, runs parallel to the ultrasound transducer and monitor edge on the screen (see Fig. 4.8b).

Characteristics of the Anterior Plane
The silhouette of the ilium proximal to the bony rim inclines towards the ultrasound transducer, that means, it tilts to the left in the right upright projection (see Fig. 4.8c and Fig. 4.9).

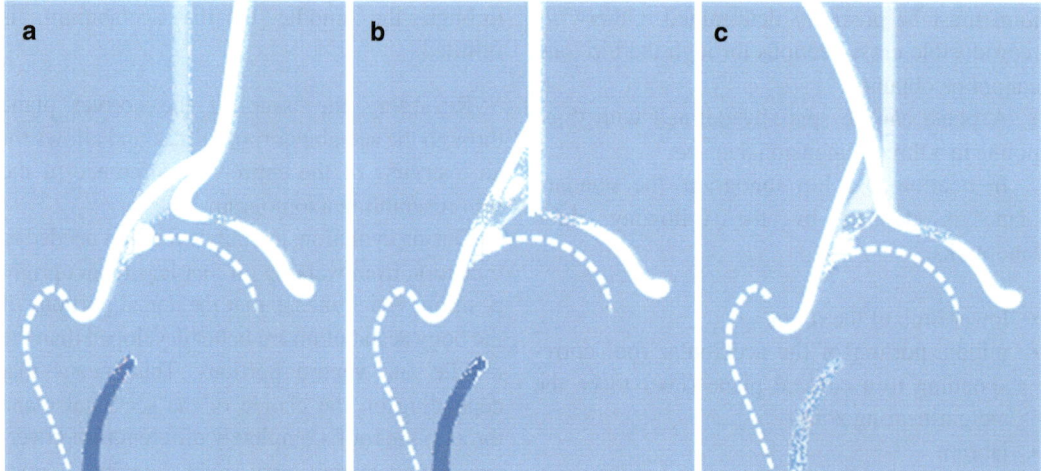

Fig. 4.8 Plane through the acetabular roof (**a**) Posterior plane. The posterior plane is characterized by a concave shape of the iliac silhouette compared to the middle plane, which has a straight iliac silhouette (see Fig. 4.8b). (**b**) Middle plane. In the middle plane, the iliac silhouette is a straight line, more or less parallel to the edge of the monitor. (**c**) Anterior plane. In the anterior plane, the iliac silhouette inclines towards the ultrasound probe, on the sonogram projecting towards the left. For comparison, the middle plane has also been outlined

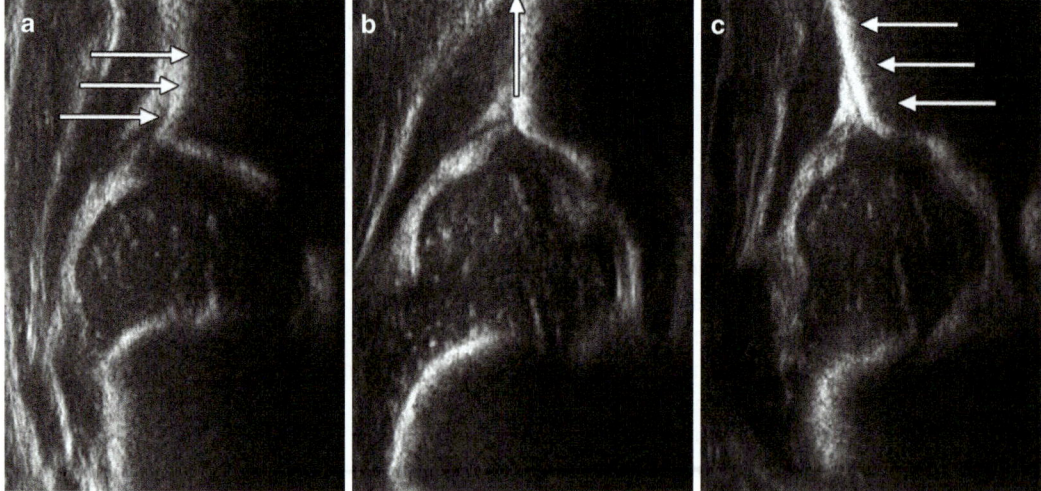

Fig. 4.9 The silhouette of the os ilium changes depending on the sectional plane. The same hip joint is shown in different sectional planes through the acetabulum. The arrows indicate the silhouette of the os ilium (**a**) posterior plane, recognizable by the concave shape of the ilium (see Fig. 4.7a2). (**b**) middle plane (standard plane) with a straight silhouette of the os ilium (see Fig. 4.7b). (**c**) anterior plane with the silhouette of the os ilium inclined towards the ultrasound transducer (see Fig. 4.7a1)

Landmark 3: Labrum

The sonographic standard plane was centred on the lower limb of the ilium and cuts through the middle section of the acetabular roof (Landmark 1; see Fig. 4.10). By aligning the plane in the middle section of the acetabular roof (Landmark 2), the bony socket is depicted (see Fig. 4.11a and Fig. 4.11b). Without the establishment of a third landmark, tilting of the plane in ventral-central and dorsal-central directions would be possible (see Fig. 4.11c). This could result in oblique

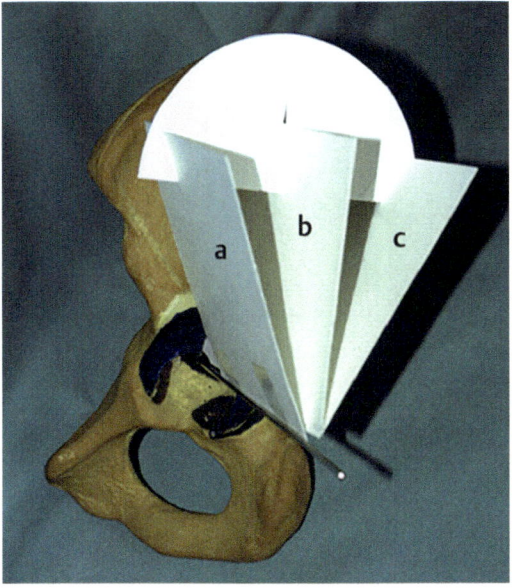

Fig. 4.10 Lower limb of the os ilium. The lower limb has been marked with a metal pin, symbolizing the axis of rotation (**a**) anterior plane (**b**) middle plane (standard plane) (**c**) posterior plane

cross sections through the hip joint, leading to subsequent distortion of the image (remember: cross-section and oblique section through a pipe). To prevent these oblique planes and tilting errors, the labrum is used as the third landmark. The labrum can only provide a clear sonographic echo if the sound beam cuts it predominantly at a perpendicular angle.

4.2.2   Usability Check

A sonogram may only be used for measurements if all the criteria of Checklist I and Checklist II are met:

- visualization of the lower limb (see Fig. 4.12).
- middle plane through the acetabular roof.
- visualization of the labrum.

Learning point
Usability checklist in short: Lower limb–Plane–Labrum.

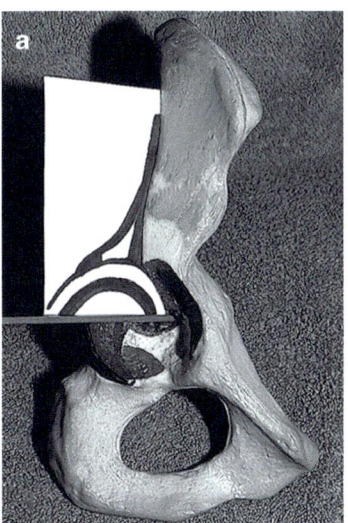
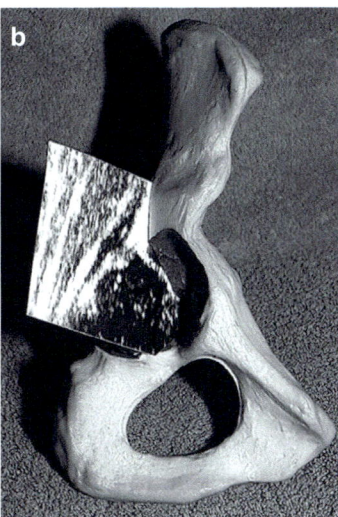
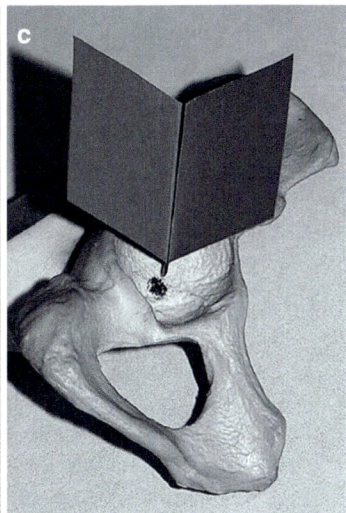

Fig. 4.11 Producing the standard (middle) plane through the acetabular roof (**a**) Diagram: The lower limb is marked with a metal pin. (**b**) The ultrasound is centred over the lower limb and the middle section of the acetabular roof.

(**c**) Oblique cuts in ventrocentral and dorsocentral directions should be avoided, as they can cause image distortion with subsequent misdiagnoses

Fig. 4.12 Presence of
the lower limb of the os
ilium. The lower limb
must be present,
otherwise the correct
plane cannot be
determined. 1 = Labrum,
2 = Lower limb. (**a**) The
lower limb is missing or
poorly defined, therefore
the sonogram is
unusable (**b**) Same hip
joint as in (**a**), the lower
limb is clearly and
distinctly visible

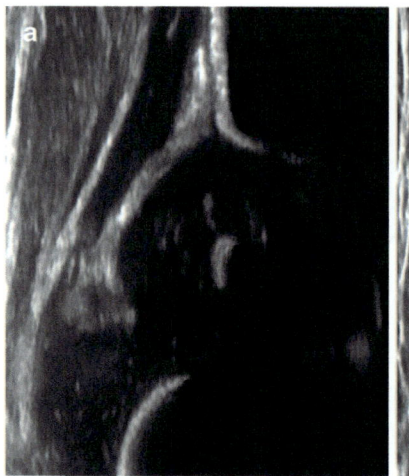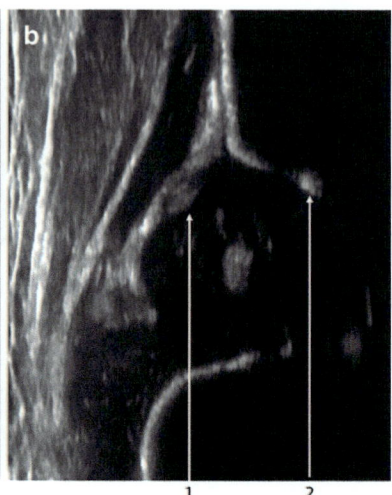

If any of these landmarks are missing, the sonogram is not usable for evaluation. Exception: in case of decentred joints, where the femoral head dislocates cranio-dorsally, the lower limb and the middle plane are often not visualized because the femoral head has moved away from the standard plane during the dislocation process.

For the reasons described above, the sequence of the usability check must be strictly followed. Very often, there is a misconception that the plane through the acetabular roof should be adjusted first. This is of no use if the lower limb is not clearly visualized first. If the lower limb is not clearly visualized, a straight silhouette of the ilium can be produced by tilting the probe, which gives the impression of being in the middle section of the acetabular roof, when this is not the case.

Practical tip
The most important step for the production of a standard plane, through the middle portion of the acetabular roof and the labrum, is to visualize the lower limb first. This is of crucial importance during the sonographic examination.

4.2.3 Checklist II

Conclusion
Checklist II: Usability Check
- Lower limb visualized?
- Middle plane visualized correctly?
- Labrum visualized?

4.2.4 Exceptions from the Standard Plane

The only exception to Checklist II occurs in dislocated joints with the femoral head dislocated cranio-dorsally and having exited the standard plane. When the femoral head slides out of the socket, it not only slides cranially but also dorsally. The dislocated femoral head and the bony socket with the lower limb then lie in different planes (Fig. 4.13).

For these dislocated hip joints, it is only important to distinguish whether the femoral head has pressed the cartilage roof upwards (Type III) or downwards (Type IV). This has implications for the classification and hip Type. With the transducer, one follows the dislocated femoral head dorsally and thus leaves the middle plane of the acetabulum (see Fig. 4.13a).

Fig. 4.13 Sectional planes in dislocated hips (**a**) The femoral head slides cranially and dorsally, thus leaving the standard plane. (**b**) Sonogram of a dislocated hip joint, Type IIIa. Due to the dorsocranial direction of dislocation, the sectional plane is dorsal. 1 = femoral head, 2 = hyaline cartilage of the acetabular roof, 3 = perichondrium going upwards, 4 = concave iliac silhouette, characteristic of the dorsal plane (**c**) Dislocated hip Type IV. The femoral head is further dislocated dorsally compared to b. This makes the concave iliac silhouette, characteristic of the dorsal plane, even more visible. The lower limb can no longer be clearly seen because the femoral head has slid out of the standard plane. 1 = femoral head, 2 = hyaline cartilage displaced downwards, 3 = tissue in the acetabular fossa, 4 = concave iliac silhouette, 5 = concave silhouette of the proximal perichondrium

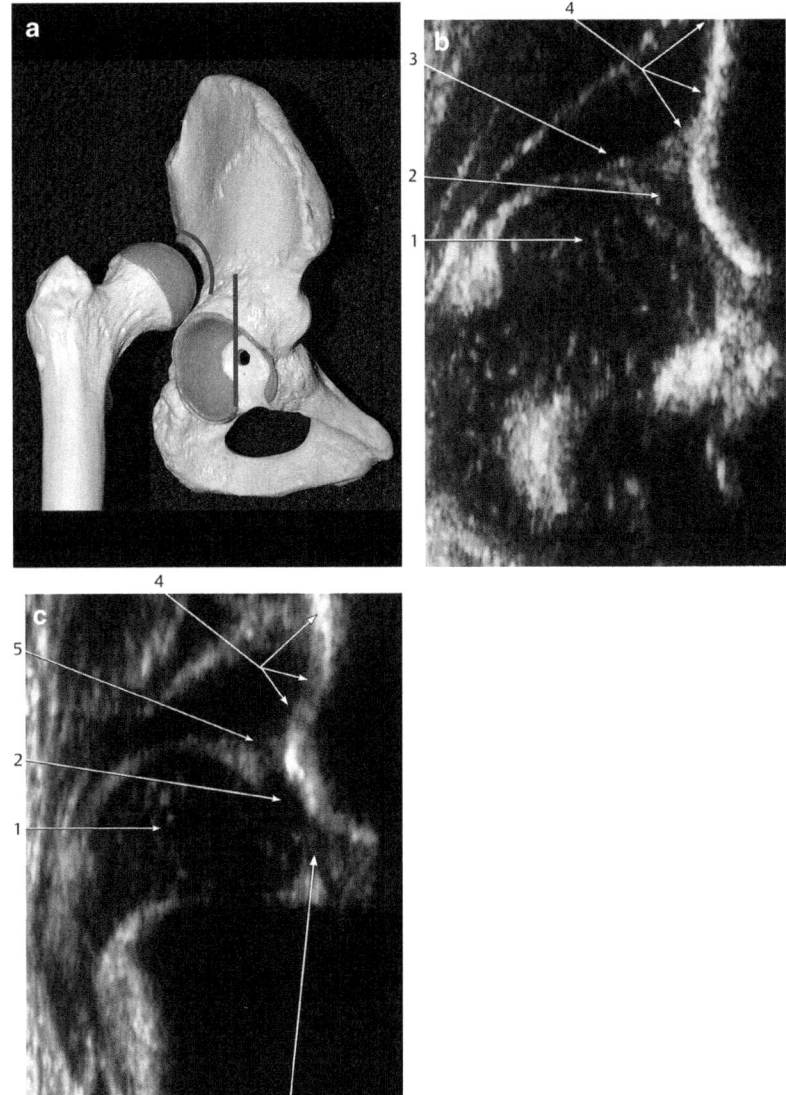

Therefore, the lower limb is often not visible and secondly, the dorsal plane is usually seen (see Fig. 4.13b and 4.13c).

4.2.5   Echoes Within the Acetabular Fossa

The anatomical structures within the acetabular fossa are reflected in a complex echo pattern. In this area, the acetabular fossa consists of three layers (see Fig. 4.14):

- Deep layer (medial layer): Consists cranially of the os ilium, dorsally of the os ischium, and ventrally of a small portion of the os pubis. All bones are connected by the triradiate cartilage (see Fig. 3.25).
- Middle layer: Consists of connective tissue and fat that line the acetabular fossa.
- Superficial layer: Consists of the ligamentum teres and the transverse ligament.

The different structures of the acetabular fossa create different echoes depending on the plane. By analysing the various planes from cranial to

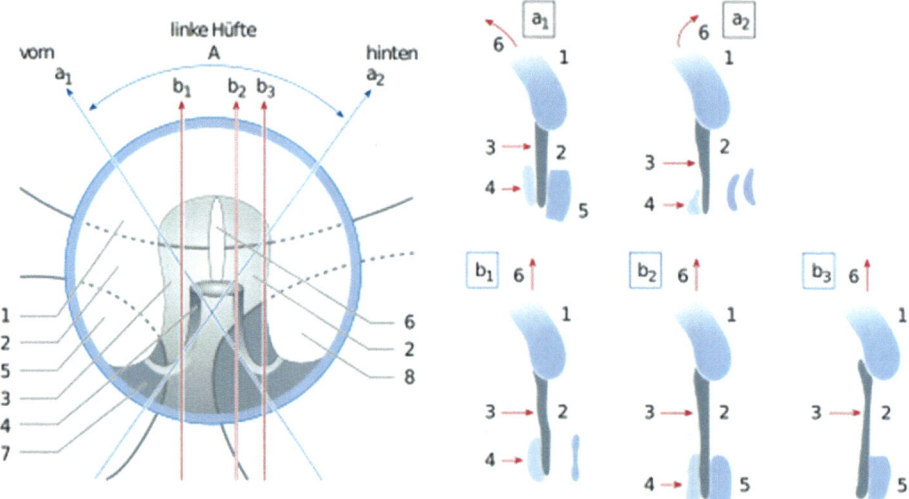

Fig. 4.14 Anatomical structures within the acetabular fossa. Left: Schematic drawing of the left acetabulum corresponding to Fig. 4.7. a1 = plane from antero-superior to dorso-inferior, a2 = plane from dorso-superior to antero-inferior, b1, b2, b3 = straight frontal planes (anterior/middle/posterior) (1 = lunate surface of the joint cartilage, 2 = horizontal part of the triradiate cartilage, 3 = tissue within the acetabular fossa, partially dissected, 4 = ligamentum teres, 5 = pubic bone covered by the lunate sur-face, 6 = cross-section of the tissue within the acetabular fossa, 7 = transverse acetabular ligament, 8 = os ischium). Right: Echoes corresponding to the planes in the left picture. a1, a2 = rotated planes, b1, b2, b3 = straight coronal planes, (1 os ilium, 2 hypoechogenic zone of the triradiate cartilage, 3 tissue in the acetabular fossa, 4 ligamentum teres, 5 ischium, 6 contours of the os ilium) (directed forward in a1, backward in a2; straight in the sectional planes b1, b2, and b3)

caudal, the anatomical structures of the acetabular fossa can be shown in different ways.

4.3   Summary

Before evaluating the hip sonogram, the anatomical identification must always be done first (Checklist I, p. 46) (Fig. 4.15a). This should be done before the usability check (Checklist II). If the usability check is done first, one of the three important landmarks could be incorrectly identified, leading to errors with potentially severe consequences. For example, confusing the lower limb of the ilium with the central fovea or mistaking the synovial fold for the labrum.

Whether a sonogram can be used for evaluation and if it meets the quality standard is decided by the usability check after the anatomical identification of all the essential echoes (p. 49). A sonogram can only be used for measurement if the femoral head is centred in the standard plane (measurement plane).

Learning points
Checklist I

Anatomical identification of the following structures:

- chondro-osseous border.
- femoral head.
- synovial fold.
- joint capsule.
- labrum.
- standard sequence (Labrum–Cartilage–Bone).
- turning point (concavity-convexity).

Checklist II

Usability check:

- Is the lower limb visible?
- Is the middle plane correct?
- Is the labrum visible?

Quick check: Lower limb–Plane–Labrum.

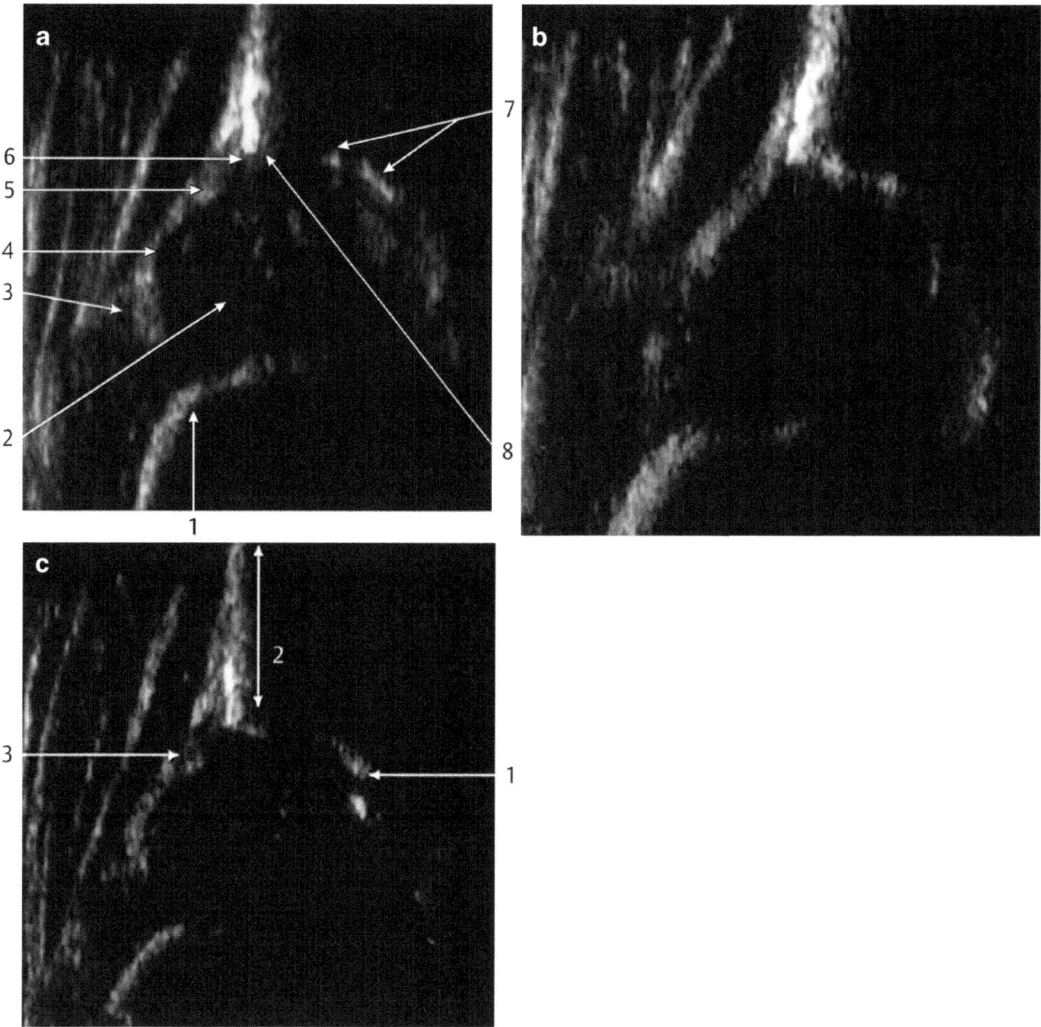

Fig. 4.15 Tactical approach to hip sonography. (**a**) Checklist I: 1 = chondro-osseous border, 2 = femoral head, 3 = synovial fold, 4 = joint capsule, 5 = labrum, 6 = hyaline cartilage roof, 7 = bony roof, 8 = turning point. (**b**) Checklist II: Is the lower limb of the ilium present? Is the plane correct? Is the labrum visible? In this example, none of the three landmarks are correctly visualized. (**c**) Same hip joint as in B, but in a different plane: the sonogram is correct. The lower limb of the ilium is accurately shown. The straight silhouette of the ilium and the labrum are visible. 1 = lower limb, 2 = silhouette of the ilium, 3 = labrum

References

1. Graf R. Kursus der Hüftsonographie beim Säugling. Stuttgart: Gustav Fischer; 1995a.

2. Graf R. Probleme und Fehlerquellen bei der Hüftsonographie. Pädiat Prax. 1995b;49:467–75.

Positioning, Scanning Technique, and Possible Errors

5

The assessment of the infant hip with sonography is independent of the position. Therefore, it is generally irrelevant how the infant is positioned. However, it has proven to be most effective to position the infant on its side and direct the sound waves in a coronal plane. The major trochanter serves as the point of contact. By following the correct procedure, it is possible to create an optimal hip sonogram in a very short time. The infant should be comfortably positioned on its side. A cradle and ultrasound probe guide are mandatory. This ensures that the baby remains as calm as possible during the examination. Any attempts to forcibly hold the baby in a fixed position during the examination, such as the accompanying person, holding the leg, should be avoided. The ultrasound should be performed before the clinical examination in order to not unsettle the baby (Fig. 5.1).

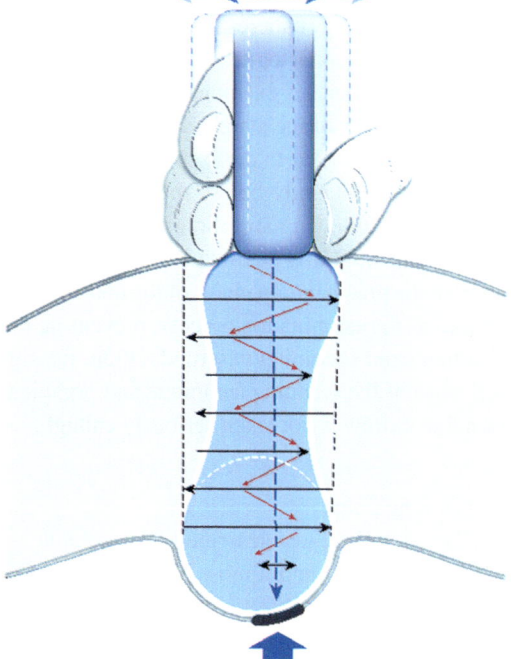

Fig. 5.1 Locating the lower limb. The vertically aligned transducer is moved forwards and backwards over the hip joint in long parallel movements to visualize the femoral head (long arrows). Afterwards, small forward and backward movements (small arrows) are used to locate the lower limb (thick arrow) then the ultrasound image is frozen

5.1   Advantages of the Recommended Examination Technique

The problem: The three landmarks, lower limb, plane, and labrum, need to be seen. These structures are only millimetres in size and often the infant is moving.

The scanning technique can be taught and learnt and is independent of the examiner's skill-set. The advantage of the recommended technique of hip sonographic examination is that it can be standardized and learnt by anyone if the instructions are strictly and correctly followed.

The importance of the time factor in the examination is usually underestimated. Every child starts moving sooner or later, making it difficult even for experienced examiners to visualize the three landmarks of the standard plane simultaneously. It is important to perform the examination quickly and efficiently before the baby becomes restless. By following specific instructions about the organization, it is possible to standardize and shorten the pre-scanning phase of the consultation as well as the examination process, preventing the children from becoming unsettled. Often, the significance of the scanning technique and organizational workflow is not taken seriously enough.

> **Learning point**
> The technique as described is teachable and learnable, and almost always guarantees a good quality of sonograms, regardless of the compliance of the accompanying person and child, as well as the experience of the examiner.

The recommended guidelines were developed based on pros and cons lists during international training courses.

5.2   Positioning the Baby

The cradle works according to the so-called hammock principle like an elastic clamp. An incontinence pad is loosely positioned over the raised edges of the cradle. The baby is placed in the hammock that is created by the pad. Depending on the size of the infant, the examiner can vary the depth of the cradle so that the hip being examined protrudes slightly over the raised edges of the cradle. For various reasons, it is recommended that the examination is performed while standing, rather than sitting (see Fig. 2.1). For this purpose, a table adapted to the height of the examiner is necessary.

> **Practical tip**
> To ensure tilt-free investigations, it is strongly recommended to use a probe guide system.

5.3   Clinic Set-up in Practice

5.3.1   Equipment

Recommendations (Fig. 5.2):

- Before entering the examination room, there should be a changing table or similar prepared so that the accompanying person can remove the nappy and, if necessary, clean the child calmly and without stress.
- In the examination room, there should also be a changing table where the child can be undressed by the parent or where the loose nappy can be removed. This table is also used for the clinical examination after the ultrasound. Handbags, paperwork, clothes, bottles, etc. that are brought along are also placed there.
- The ultrasound machine, if possible with a foot pedal, is positioned to the right side of the examiner.

5.3.2   Position of the Examiner and the Accompanying Adult

The examiner stands in a position where their right hand is near the head of the baby, while the accompanying person stands on the other side of the cradle (see Fig. 2.1). This allows the examiner to

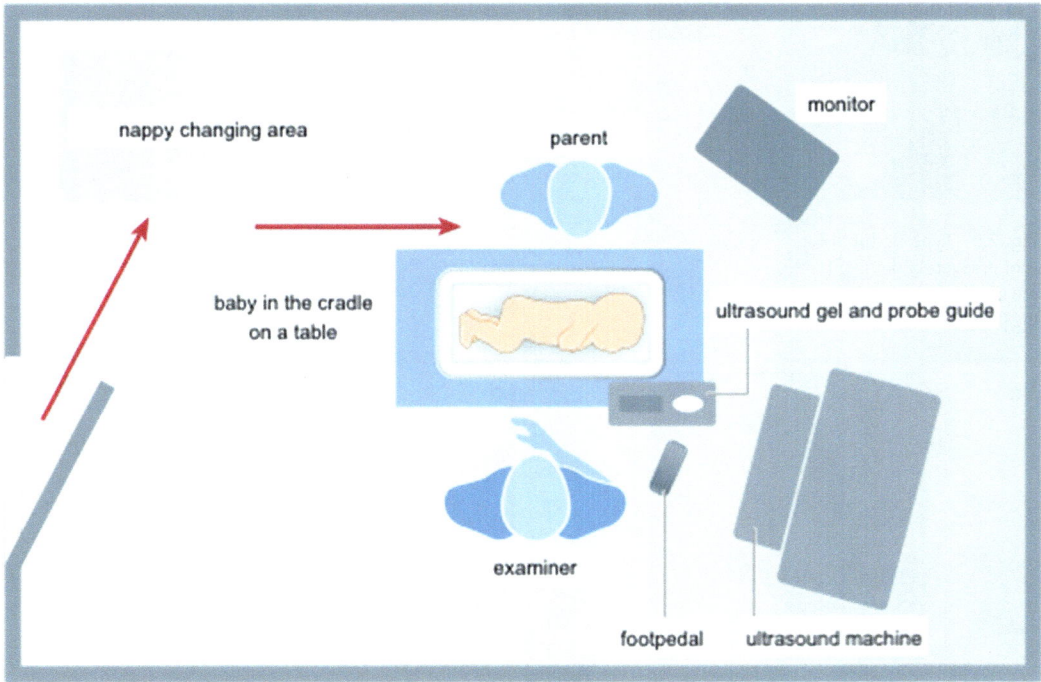

Fig. 5.2 Equipment required for hip ultrasound. Organizational adaptations in practice. In some cases, an additional monitor to rotate the image can also be used

examine comfortably from the side and rest their forearms on the edge of the cradle without having to contort their body. This enables smooth guidance of the ultrasound probe. Additionally, when placing the baby on its side, it is important to ensure that the legs are not pulled by the examiner or the accompanying person in an attempt to assist, even if done in good faith. Doing so always results in a slight external rotation of the hip joint. This position and fixation not only irritate the baby and agitates them, but also causes the ultrasound probe to slip either dorsally or ventrally from the greater trochanter, which serves as the coupling point.

> **Learning point**
> It is much easier to maintain the position that the infant assumes spontaneously, rather than to try and manipulate the leg.

The slightly flexed hip and knee in a spontaneous position, do not interfere with the examination process. Slight internal rotation that occurs when the knee joint does not protrude

beyond the side of the cradle (Fig. 5.3a), rotates the greater trochanter from dorsal to ventral into the coronal plane. This eliminates the physiological anteversion through internal rotation. Thus, the greater trochanter, the femoral neck, and the acetabulum are aligned in one plane (Fig. 5.3b).

5.3.3 Instructions and Guidance to the Accompanying Adult

The accompanying adults are often nervous. Clear instructions help reduce organizational chaos, radiate calmness, and build trust. The following recommendations and behaviour may seem silly, but they have been developed and proven to be excellent over many years:

- All personal data should already be entered into the US machine before the parent enters the examination room with the child.
Remember:
- The examiner stands by the examination table and greets the person entering: "Hello, Mr/

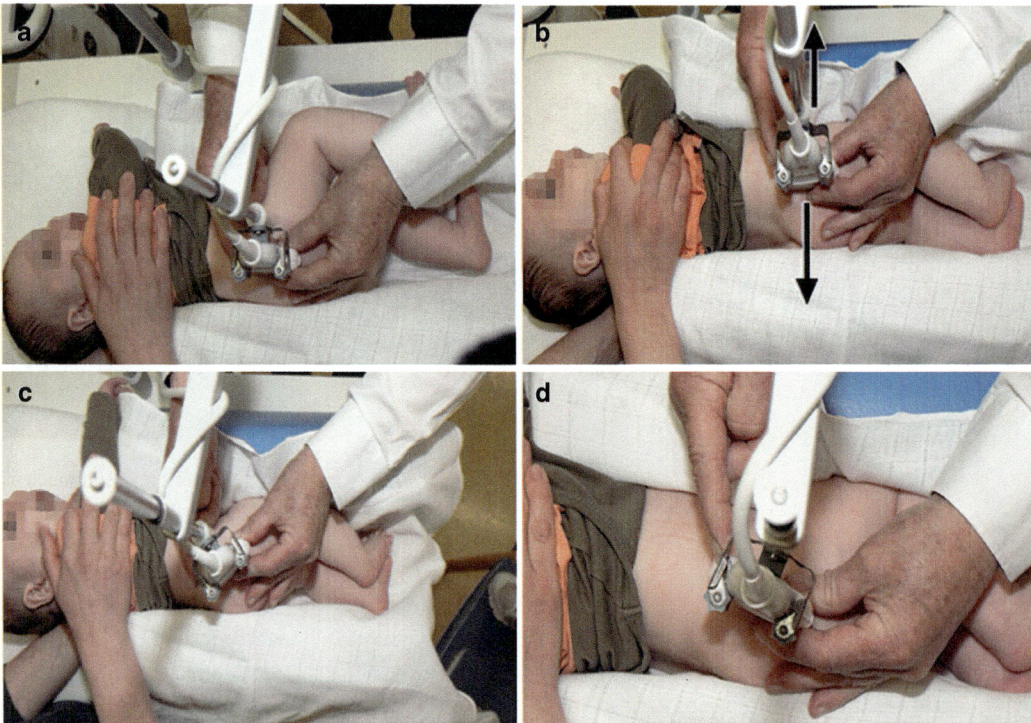

Fig. 5.3 Positioning and scanning technique. View from the top (**a**) Incorrect positioning and scanning technique. The leg slides over the bolster and moves forward. The greater trochanter rotates slightly dorsally, making the scanning process more difficult. (**b**) Correct positioning and scanning technique. The leg is slightly internally rotated, and the knee does not slide over the bolster of the cradle. The image shows the starting position with the ultrasound probe placed straight and perpendicular over the baby's hip. The arrows mark the movements of the probe: By moving the left hand forward and backward, the lower limb of the ilium is visualized, and the sonogram is frozen regardless of the plane. (**c**) Plane over the posterior part of the acetabulum (hip socket). (**d**) Plane over the anterior part of the acetabulum

Mrs. M." The accompanying adult often has no free hand and is forced to put their baby in an awkward position to shake hands with the doctor. Therefore, it is best to limit the greeting to a verbal one.

- The examiner points out the provided changing table with the instruction: "Please lay your child on the table and, if necessary, remove the nappy also, put down your bag".
- The examiner points to the opposite side of the cradle with the request: "Please come over here and give me your child".
- Important: The examiner takes the child from the accompanying person and lays it sideways in the cradle, so that the right hip joint can be examined first. The accompanying person should not place the child in the cradle themselves, as the position is often incorrect.

Turning the baby around confuses and irritates it.

- The examination should start with the right hip joint, as the child is distracted by the ultrasound machine lights on the right side.
- The examiner gives the accompanying person the following instruction: "Please place your right hand on the (right) shoulder of the child".

Practical tip
- The accompanying adult should be involved in the examination process and stay with the child.
- It is important that the accompanying adult holds the child's shoulder and not their wrist and does not grip or restrain

them (Fig. 5.4). Restricting the movement of older children can provoke defensive reactions.

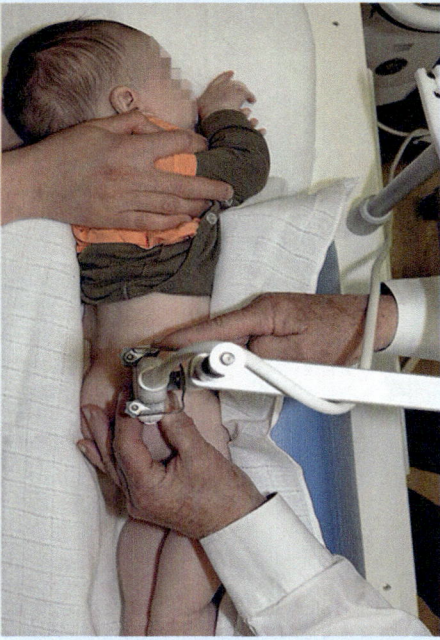

Fig. 5.4 Instructions to the accompanying person. The child is lying in the cradle. The hand of the accompanying person is correctly placed on the child's shoulder. The ultrasound probe is placed parallel to the bolsters of the cradle and perpendicular to the hip joint; the fingers are correctly placed (extended); the middle and index fingers guide the ultrasound probe. The index finger of the right hand stabilizes the transducer and rotates it to adjust the desired view

- The positioning should be in a natural position, with legs slightly bent. Under no circumstances should the accompanying adult or examiner pull or stretch the child's legs. This would only lead to defensive movements.

5.4   Scanning Technique

5.4.1   Right Hip Joint

Adopting the correct position

- Step 1: The left hand rests on the baby's right leg and slightly rotates it inward so that the knee joint is in the cradle and does not protrude beyond the bolster.
- Step 2: The gel is applied to the skin, not the transducer, so that the examiner's fingers can immediately feel the trochanter through a sliding motion.
- Step 3:
  - Finger position: The left thumb is placed at the front and with the extended middle and index fingers of the left hand placed in the gel on the greater trochanter (see Fig. 5.4). Fingers IV and V are slightly spread apart from the other fingers.
  - Transducer position: The transducer is now placed parallel to the bolsters of the cradle and perpendicular to the greater trochanter using the right hand (not turned towards the spine and not tilted; see Fig. 5.4).
  - The fingertips of the left hand, lying on the greater trochanter are pushed apart by the probe.
  - The fingers should not be flexed, as this may cause the fingernails to touch child's skin and provoke defensive reactions (see Fig. 5.5).

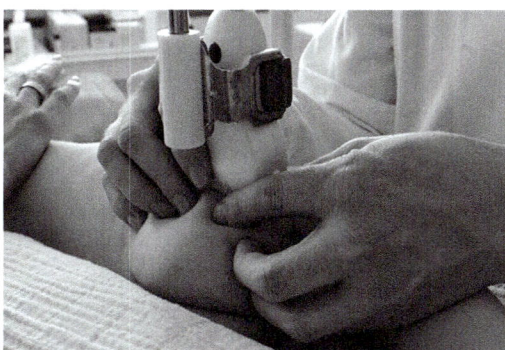

Fig. 5.5 Incorrect hand and transducer position. The fingers of the left hand are flexed, and the fingernails irritate the infant by applying pressure on the skin

- Step 4:
  - Finger position of the right hand: The index finger is extended while the other fingers are holding the thumb (see Fig. 5.4).
  - Both wrists are supported on the bolsters of the cradle. Pay attention to the right forearm: it should also rest on the bolsters of the cradle.

Practical tip

Before the examiner looks at the monitor, he/she must visually check the position of the fingers, the hands, and the transducer:

- Fingers: The thumb is placed in front, the middle and index fingers are placed behind the transducer, so that it is gripped in a clamp-like manner. The fingers are straight, the middle finger touches the transducer and the child.
- Transducer: It is vertical and aligned parallel to the bolsters of the cradle.
- Hand: Both forearms are supported on the bolsters of the cradle.

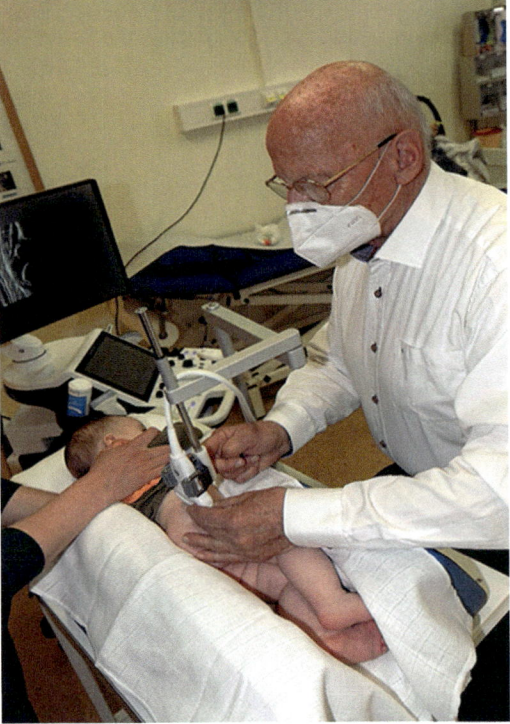

Fig. 5.6 Third step of the examination: plane correction. The plane is corrected by rotating around the central axis of the ultrasound probe using the index finger of the right hand under direct vision

Image Acquisition

Note: First, the joint must be seen in the standard plane (Checklist I).

To make a diagnosis, Checklist II is then followed.

- Step 1:
  - The transducer is moved back and forth over the hip joint, parallel to the cradle and starting from the position described above, in order to visualize the round shape of the femoral head.
  - The index finger of the right hand stabilizes the transducer to prevent it from rotating during the parallel movements.
- Main movements to visualize the lower limb:
  - forward - backward - forward - backward (Where is the joint?)
  - smaller - smaller - smaller - stop (Where is the lower limb?).

- Step 3:
  - While looking at the frozen sonogram, the examiner calmly orients themselves on the plane and considers in which direction the transducer may need to be rotated (ventral or dorsal; see Fig. 5.3c and Fig. 5.3d). The extent of the rotation is estimated.
  - The rotation is now performed in the desired direction, with the index finger of the right hand while the finger position of the left hand remains unchanged, with the transducer over the trochanter.
  - Keyword: readjustment (see Fig. 5.6).
  - The examiner now looks at the monitor.
  - Movement: forward - backward - forward - backward (see Fig. 5.1, Fig. 5.3b).
- Step 2:
  - Once the entire hip joint is identified, focus on the lower limb of the ilium. Since this

area is very small, the parallel movements are also smaller.

- Once the lower limb is captured through tiny movements, the ultrasound image is immediately frozen ignoring all other structures.
- Movement: smaller - smaller - smaller - stop.
- Step 4: The examiner looks back from the transducer to the monitor, searches for the lower limb by parallel movements as in steps 1 and 2 and freezes the picture again.
- Step 5:
  - Once the lower limb is visualised, the picture is frozen, the plane is then checked again. If the plane is correct, the examination process is usually finished as all other structures in checklists I and II, including the labrum, are captured automatically with this scanning technique.
  - If the plane is not correct, further readjustment (rotation) is performed and the lower limb is again found by parallel movements.

Practical tip
Mnemonic for scanning technique:

- forward-backward-forward-backward,
- smaller - smaller - smaller - stop
- rotate
- forward-backward-forward-backward, smaller - smaller - smaller - stop

Learning point
When performing the sectional plane correction (rotation), it is important to look at the ultrasound probe to avoid unintentional tilting.

5.4.2 Left Hip Joint

Repositioning the Child and Assuming the Examination Position
The child is turned onto its left side in the cradle by the examiner not the accompanying person after examining the right hip joint: The examiner's left hand grasps the child's ankles, while the right hand gently pulls on the left arm. By supinating the examiners left hand, a rotational movement is created, allowing the child to be turned over in the cradle without having to lift it out. The accompanying person's hand is immediately placed back on the child's shoulder (see Fig. 5.7).

Image Acquisition
- Step 1:
  - The left hand of the examiner is placed flat on the left hip joint, with the trochanter palpable between the thumb and index finger.
  - The forearm of the examiner rests lightly on the child's leg, with the remaining fingertips resting on the bolster of the cradle. This prevents the leg from sliding out and allows for a slight internal rotation.
  (see Fig. 5.7b).
- Step 2:
  - The transducer is held in a similar way to the right hip joint, but this time only resting between the thumb and index finger.
  - The transducer is again positioned perpendicular and parallel to the bolster of the cradle.
  - The index finger of the right hand stabilizes the ultrasound probe and rotates it in the desired direction.

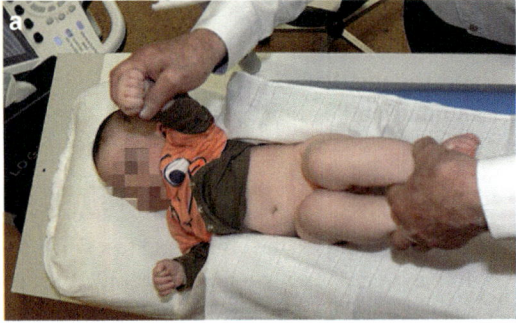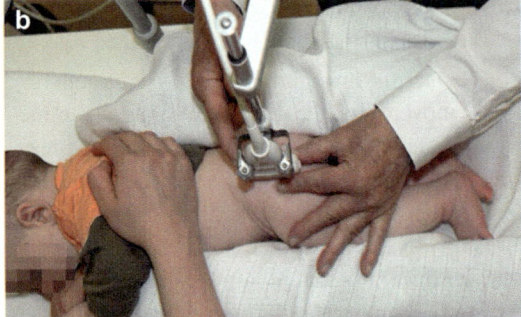

Fig. 5.7 Repositioning of the child by the examiner (**a**) With careful traction on the legs and left arm, the rotation of the child is achieved without lifting it out of the hammock. (**b**) Starting position for the examination of the left hip joint. Defining the examination area by feeling for the trochanter with the thumb and index finger and placement of the probe without tilting. At the same time, with the left hand, the leg is gently internally rotated to prevent the leg from sliding out of the cradle. The parent stabilizes the child's shoulder with their hand

- Step 3:
  - forward - backward - forward - backward, etc. (finding the lower limb).
  - rotate.
  - forward - backward - forward - backward, etc. - stop.

5.5   Summary

Conclusion
- **Preparation:**
  - Perform examination while standing.
  - Guide the accompanying person verbally and non-verbally through gestures.
- **"Intermezzo":**
  - Take the child from the accompanying person and position it in the cradle, starting with the right hip joint.
  - Place the accompanying person's right hand on the child's right shoulder.
  - Slightly internally rotate the leg.
  - Apply gel on the child's skin.
  - Eye contact: Finger - transducer - hand.

- **Examination Technique:`**
  - Forward-backward-forward-backward, etc.
- (Visualization of the lower limb)
  - Rotate (correct the plane while looking at the transducer).
  - Forward-backward-forward-backward, etc. (again visualize the lower limb and check the plane).
  - Change position for examination of the left hip:
  - Pay attention to the altered hand position, forward - backward - forward - backward, etc.

5.6   Possible Sources of Error

5.6.1   Problems Related to the Organization and to the Position

- There is no changing table prepared, which distresses the child when being undressed. The examination is carried out while sitting. Consequences: there is a loss of time until the examiner and accompanying person are positioned, the examiner sits in a twisted manner.

- The examiner approaches the examination table from the wrong side. This is important because the right and left hand of the examiner have different tasks: the more skilled right hand (for right-handed individuals) takes control of the transducer for adjusting the standard plane.
- The accompanying person has no opportunity to clean their child in peace and quiet before entering the examination room. If the child is undressed in the examination room, it can become restless.
- The child is fed to calm it during the examination; this only shows a lack of scanning technique. If the child needs to be calmed down, feeding should be done at an appropriate gap before the examination.
- The gel is warmed up and liquifies as a result. The infant is not distressed by gel at room temperature, but rather by incorrect handling and incorrect scanning technique.
- The legs are stretched (Fig. 5.8), and the child is fixed by the wrists. This provokes defensive reactions.
- The transducer is tilted towards the spine, and the fingers are flexed rather than extended. The angled ultrasound beam causes tilting errors (p. 67). The flexed fingers provoke the baby's defensive reactions due to uncomfortable pressure (see Fig. 5.5).
- Attempts are made to visualize the lower limb through rotating and tilting movements (called "brushing"). However, this technique does not clearly demarcate the lower limb from the surrounding tissues.
- Correction of the plane is attempted through uncontrolled rotating and tilting movements while looking at the monitor. However, this often results in the loss of the lower limb.

Note: left-handers are advised to proceed with a mirrored scanning technique.

> **Note**
> A semi-automatic, computer-assisted examination technique is under development. The prototype is promising and results in excellent image quality in a very short examination time.

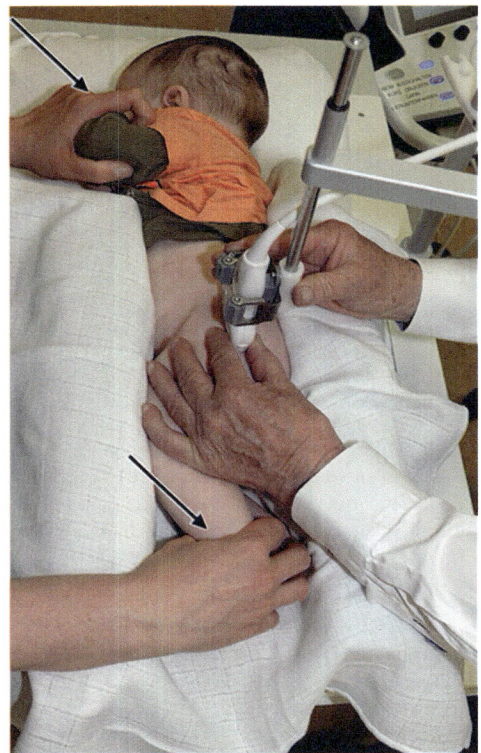

Fig. 5.8 Incorrect hand position of the parent. In case of a restless baby, the child in this example is reflexively pushed down (top arrow). The accompanying person pulls on the leg (lower arrow), thereby straightening the hip and knee joints. This causes defensive reactions and movements by the baby. Additionally, the slight internal rotation of the hip joint is eliminated by this movement. The position of the examiner's right hand is incorrect. Only the index finger of the right hand should be used to adjust the plane

5.6.2   Tilting Errors

Due to tilting of the ultrasound probe and subsequent oblique direction of ultrasound waves entering the hip joint, there are typical distortions of the image caused by the different sound velocities in the cartilage, muscles, and bones due to refraction and diffraction of the sound beam.

Tilt in ventro-dorsal direction
This direction of the sound beam, causes a poorly defined widening of the echoes of the proximal perichondrium and the ilium, making it difficult to correctly assess the ilium and draw the baseline (p. 74) (Fig. 5.9).

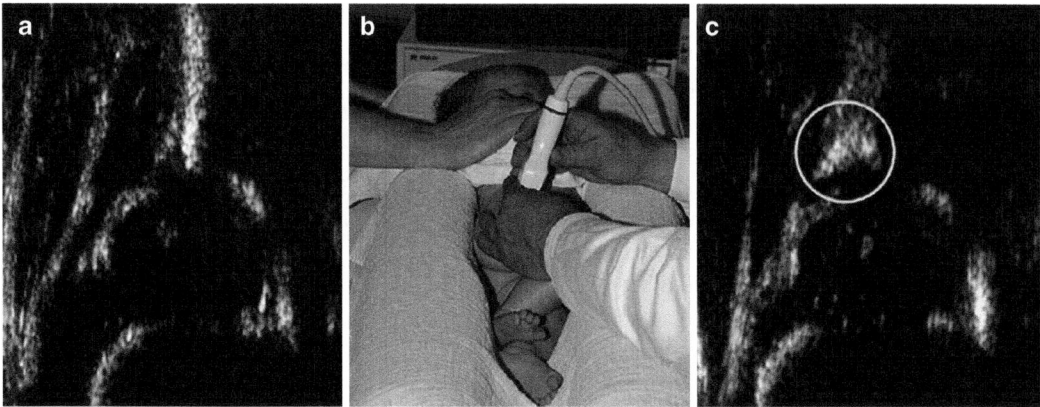

Fig. 5.9 Tilting in ventro-dorsal direction (**a**) Correct ultrasound scan without tilting errors. (**b**) Tilting of the ultrasound probe in ventro-dorsal direction. (**c**) Ultrasound scan with ventro-dorsal tilt, identifiable by the widening of the proximal perichondrium (circle) and the relative blurriness of the iliac silhouette. For comparison, see the correct ultrasound scan in (**a**)

Fig. 5.10 Tilting in the dorso-ventral direction (**a**) Tilting of the ultrasound probe in the dorso-ventral direction. (**b**) Sonogram with dorso-ventral tilt. The tilting can be seen in the concave iliac silhouette, corresponding to the dorsal section. Compare correct sonogram in Fig. 5.9a

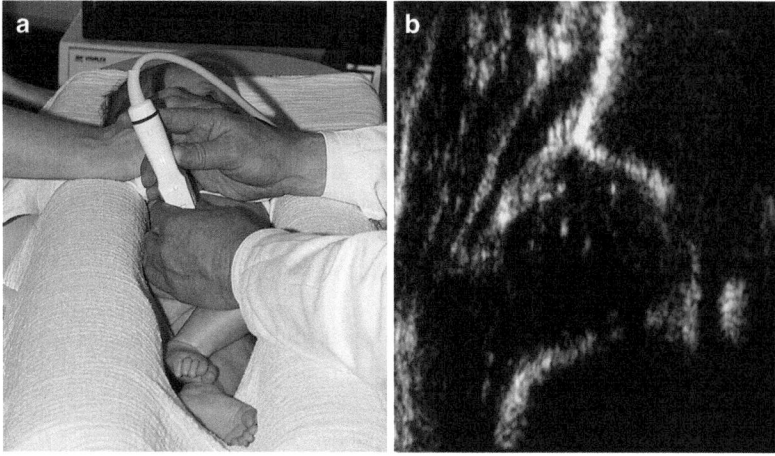

Tilt in the dorso-ventral direction

With this direction of tilt, the plane displayed appears dorsal (Fig. 5.10). The concavity of the ilium is created by the fact that the sound beam hits the gluteal fossa. To the surprise of the examiner, this apparent dorsal plane does not disappear even when the transducer is rotated further ventrally if the tilt is not corrected.

Tilt in a cranio-caudal direction

In this tilting mistake, the lower edge of the iliac bone is often not seen because the cranio-caudally directed ultrasound beam is blocked by the ilium (Fig. 5.11).

Tilt in a caudo-cranial direction

This is the most serious of all the tilting errors (Fig. 5.12). Due to caudo-cranial tilting of the ultrasound probe, the ultrasound beam is bent, refracted, and reflected at the different boundary surfaces. As a result, the middle portion of the acetabulum can appear to be a dorsal plane. If an attempt is made to visualize the central plane by rotating the probe ventrally, anatomically speaking, one is then in the ventral area of the acetabulum. Additionally, the femoral head usually takes on a more elongated shape and the chondro-osseous border becomes increasingly less visible. The bony socket appears flattened and is poorly

Fig. 5.11 Tilt in
cranio-caudal direction
(**a**) Tilt of the ultrasound
probe in cranio-caudal
direction. (**b**) Sonogram
with cranio-caudal tilt.
The lower limb can no
longer be shown
accurately. Compare the
correct sonogram in
Fig. 5.9a

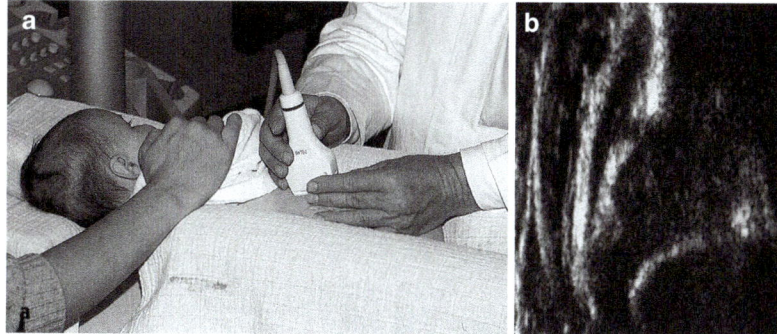

Fig. 5.12 Tilt in
caudo-cranial direction
(**a**) Tilting of the
ultrasound probe in
caudo-cranial direction.
(**b**) Sonogram with
caudo-cranial tilt. Due to
differences in
propagation time,
diffraction and
refraction, image
distortion occurs. The
caudo-cranial beam
direction is recognized
by the almost complete
disappearance of the
chondro-osseous border.
In **b**, the hip joint
appears significantly
worse than in **c**. (**c**)
Correct sonogram

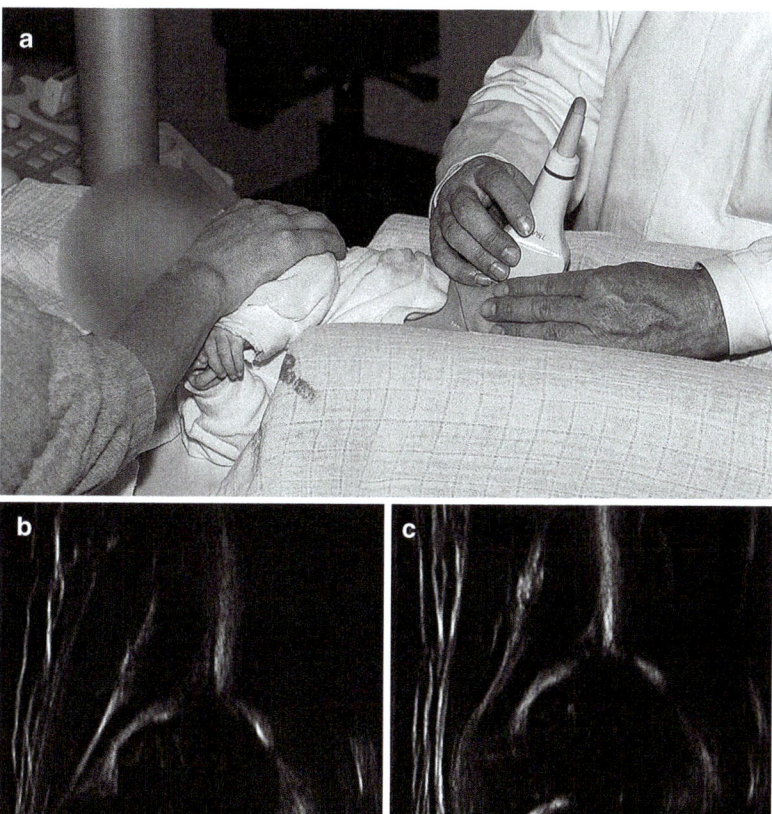

defined, leading to over-diagnosis due to the apparent pathological findings.

Practical Tip
- A straight beam direction is required for the examination. Sector scanners should not be used. A probe guide is indispensable, which only allows the movements important for scanning but blocks all the other unwanted movements.
- Sonograms without a chondro-osseous border should not be used for diagnosis. If the chondro-osseous border is visible, the caudo-cranial tilting error, which leads to over-diagnosis, is largely excluded (see also Checklist I).

Measurement Techniques and Possible Sources of Errors

6

6.1   Angle Measurement

The system for angle measurements, which is currently used worldwide, is established for over 30 years. It has been shown in daily practice to be superior to all other systems. Attempts to introduce additional angles or ratios (Harcke, Terjesen, Suzuki) beyond the bony α angle and cartilage β angle [1] have not improved the precision of this measurement system. Measurement systems that, for diagnosis, use the centre of the hip joint and percentages of head coverage or the distance of the femoral head (simulated as a circle on the computer) from the bony acetabular fossa, do not meet modern standards expected today.

The advantage of the system of angle measurement is that the proportions of the acetabular roof and the ratio of cartilage to bone remain the same regardless the size of the hip joint being measured. The biomechanical conditions also remain identical.

The definitions of the measurement lines have been adapted for sonographic practice and do not conform to the conventional mathematical definitions of a line. The two angles formed by the measurement lines characterize the shape of the bony socket with the bony roof angle α and the shape of the cartilaginous roof with the cartilage roof angle β. Using these two angles, the overall shape of the bony and cartilaginous parts of the acetabulum can, in centred joints, be assigned a type.

Learning point
Developmental hip dysplasia is a pathology of the acetabulum. The measurement system with α and β angles has the advantage of being independent of the position of the leg and the femoral head.

6.2   Bony Roof Line

6.2.1   Definition

The echo of the lower limb represents a pivot point from which a line is drawn laterally tangential to the echo of the bony roof (see Fig. 6.1a). This definition is applicable whether the bony rim, the most lateral part of the bony acetabulum, is angular, rounded, or flattened.

Note
For practical reasons, the definition of the bony roof line is "tangential to the bony roof," not "tangential to the turning point."

R. Graf et al., *Sonography of the Infant's Hip*, https://doi.org/10.1007/978-3-031-71949-3_6

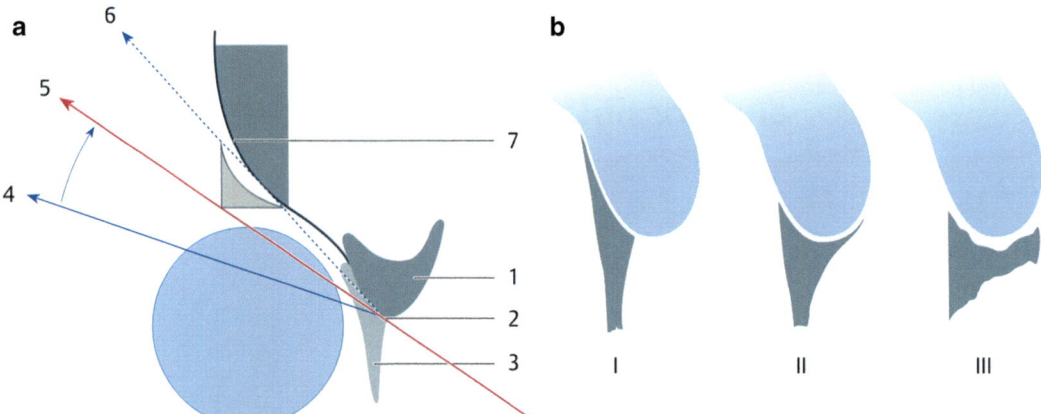

Fig. 6.1 Bony roof line (**a**) The bony roof line is placed tangential to, touching, the echo of the bony socket pivoting from the edge of the lower limb (1 = os ilium, 2 = lower limb of the os ilium, 3 = fatty connective tissue in the acetabular fossa, 4 = start of the bony roof line at the pivot point (lower limb), 5 = bony roof line with an angular bony rim, 6 = bony roof line with a rounded bony rim, 7 = rounded bony rim) (**b**) Lower limb with surrounding echo patterns of various anatomical structures. (I = classical shape, II = chalice shape, III = "frayed" type)

6.2.2   Measurement Errors

Measurement errors usually arise from unclear or incorrect identification of the lower limb in the sonogram. The anatomy explains this error:

Area of the lower limb:

- Caudal to the lower limb, there is the triradiate cartilage, which gives sinusoidal echoes directly caudal to the lower limb, creating a fringed or cloudy appearance. These echoes must be cut off by the measurement line. Attention: The measurement line starts at the bottom of the lower limb and not in the centre of the echo (see Fig. 6.1).
- Lateral to the lower limb in the acetabular fossa, there is connective tissue. Depending on the machine setting, this can form different echoes: classic, cup-shaped, or fringed (see Fig. 6.1b) [2].
- Further lateral, between the femoral head and the fatty connective tissue, the fibres of the ligamentum teres are sometimes visible, as well as the stronger, spot-like echo of the central fovea. The connective tissue in the acetabular fossa and the echoes of the central fovea should not be confused with the lower limb (Fig. 6.2b, Fig. 6.3).

The Bony Roof
Bony Rim Defect

Ossification defects can occur in the lateral aspect of the bony roof (Fig. 6.4). These are not of any biomechanical significance unless the bony roof angle α is in the pathological range.

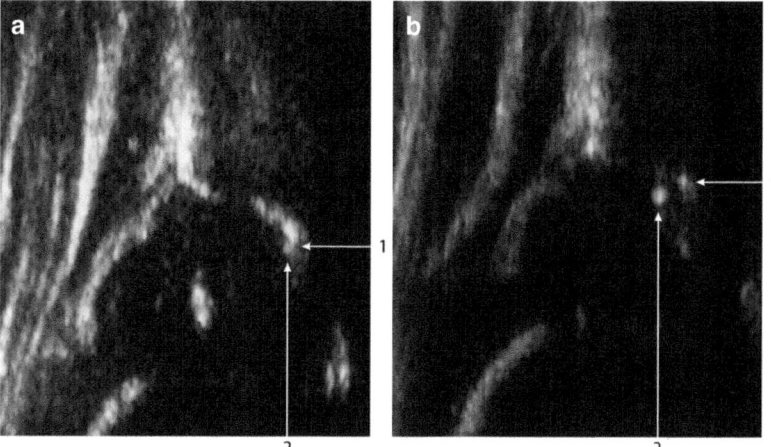

Fig. 6.2 Demarcation of the lower limb (**a**) Demarcation of the lower limb from the fatty connective tissue in the acetabular fossa (1 = lower limb, 2 = fatty connective tissue of the acetabular fossa) (**b**) Possibility of confusion with a poorly defined lower limb between the lower limb and the central fovea (1 = lower limb, 2 = central fovea as the attachment area of the ligamentum teres)

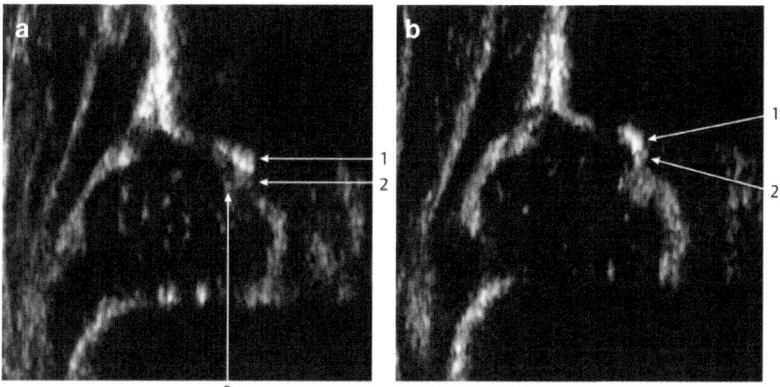

Fig. 6.3 Demarcation of the lower limb of the os ilium (**a**) Demarcation of the lower limb from the fatty connective tissue of the acetabular fossa with the ligamentum teres (1 = lower limb of the os ilium, 2 = fatty connective tissue of the acetabular fossa, 3 = ligamentum teres) (**b**) Example for the demarcation of the lower limb (see Fig. 6.1 No. 2) (1 = lower limb of the os ilium, 2 = sinusoids)

Fig. 6.4 Bony rim defect (**a**) bony rim defect laterally in the bony rim marked with an arrow. (**b**) correctly drawn measurement lines

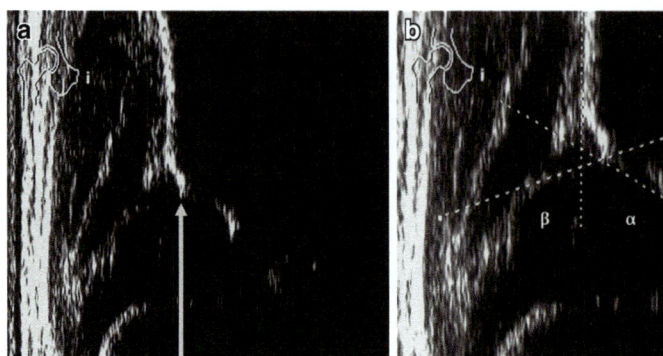

6.3   Baseline

6.3.1 Definition

An essential point for drawing the baseline is the most cranial point or Z-point (Fig. 6.5; see also Fig. 6.4b) [3]. The most cranial point (Z-point) in the sonogram is the point at which the upper portion of the echo of the proximal perichondrium comes into contact with the os ilium. However, anatomically, this is not the upper end of the hyaline cartilage acetabular roof, but the point of origin of the rectus tendon. Starting from the most cranial point as the pivot point, the baseline is drawn distally tangential to, just touching, the lateral echo of the os ilium.

Note: From the Z-point as the pivot point, the baseline is drawn distally tangential to, just touching, the lateral echo of the os ilium.

6.3.2 Problems

The most cranial point of the bony rim, which is necessary as a starting point for the baseline, sometimes cannot be found. Often this is the case, because ossification has already taken place, or because echoes have occurred between the proximal perichondrium and the ilium due to poor machine settings, making it impossible to locate this measurement point.

With a lateral sound beam, the sound wave is blocked by the os ilium and there is an acoustic shadow medial to the os ilium. The transition from an echo-rich to an echo-poor zone seems to represent the end of the cortex. The line so produced is an artefact. However, as it is formed by the sound wave being blocked at the outer cortex it therefore runs parallel to the outer cortex and thus to the original baseline. This line is referred to as the "auxiliary baseline" (see Fig. 6.5b).

Remember
Between the baseline and the bony roof line lies angle α, which is the measurement for the bony roof.

Fig. 6.5 Baseline (**a**) drawing the baseline from the most cranial point of the bony roof, touching the silhouette of the iliac bone, tangential to the echo of the ilium. (**b**) ultrasound image with auxiliary baseline drawn

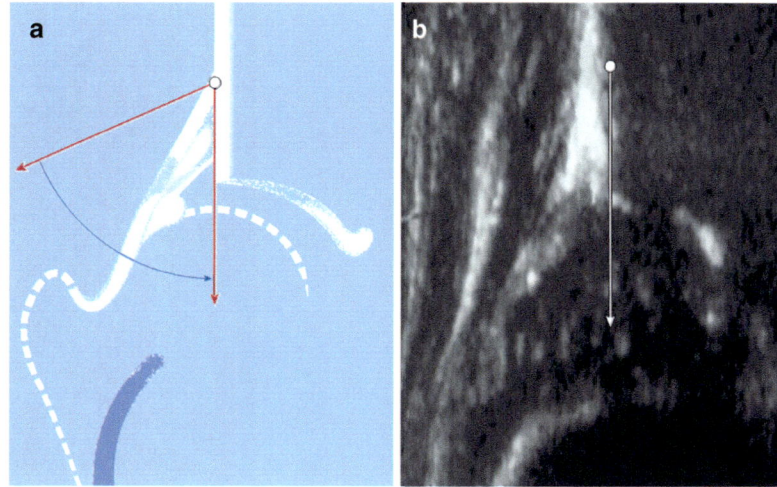

6.4   Cartilage Roof Line

6.4.1   Definition

The cartilage roof line is drawn between the turning point and the centre of the labrum (Fig. 6.6a). The cartilage roof angle β characterizes the cartilaginous part of the acetabular roof.

6.4.2   Measurement Errors

At the Turning Point
The turning point is the point where the concavity of the acetabulum turns into the convexity from caudal to cranial and is the most lateral point of the acoustic shadow (Fig. 6.6b). If one tries to determine the turning point from cranial to caudal along the echo of the bone, the turning point is usually placed incorrectly, i.e. too far cranially (Fig. 6.8a).

Caution
The turning point is rarely the intersection point of the baseline and bony roof line.

The baseline, bony roof line, and the cartilaginous roof line do not usually intersect at the same point (Fig. 6.7). This is only the case for type I joints with an angulated bony rim.

The Labrum
Unfortunately, even with high-resolution machines and good machine settings, the tip of the labrum is not always identifiable and is not suitable as a measurement point. Therefore, this has been abandoned and the centre, main echo, of the labrum has been defined as the second measurement point.

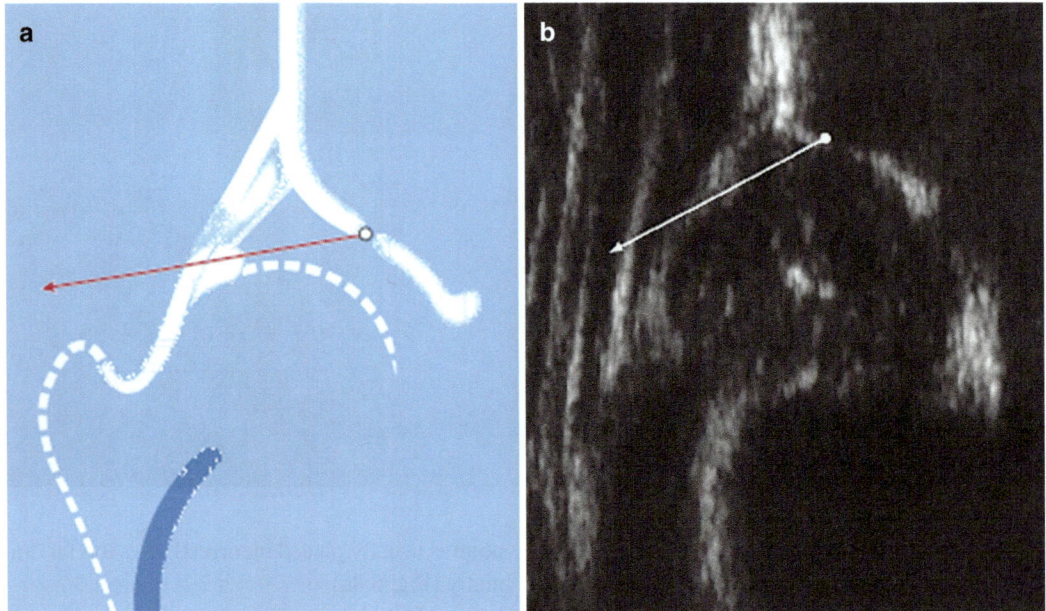

Fig. 6.6 Cartilage roof line (**a**) The cartilage roof line is the line drawn between the turning point (concavity to convexity) to The centre of the labrum. (**b**) Cartilage roof line from the most lateral point of the acoustic shadow

Fig. 6.7 Cartilage roofline (**a**) An example with correctly and incorrectly drawn cartilage roofline with the turning point incorrectly identified. (**b**) The three measurement lines with the bony roof angle α and the cartilage roof angle β correctly drawn

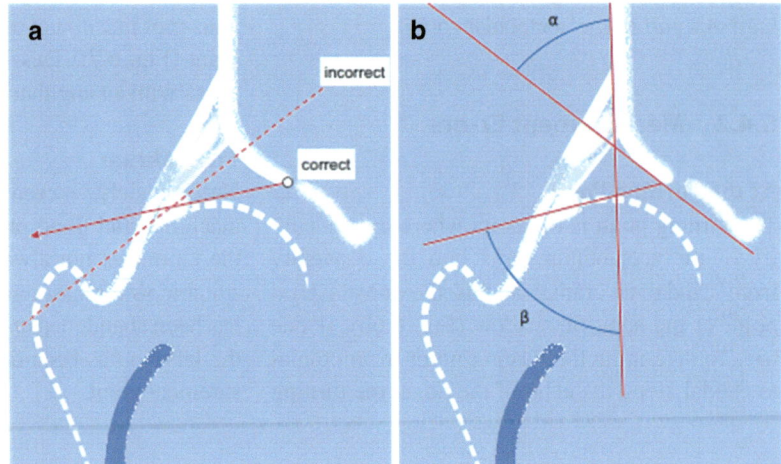

6.5 Bony Roof Angle α and Cartilage Roof Angle β

Between the bony roof line and the baseline or auxiliary baseline is the bony roof angle α, which measures the development of the bony socket. The baseline and cartilage roof line enclose the cartilage roof angle β. This is a measure of the size and shape of the cartilaginous socket which is an important factor in the development and function of the hip joint. (Fig. 6.7b and Fig. 6.8)

Fig. 6.8 Cartilage roof line and bony roof line (**a**) An example of a correctly and an incorrectly drawn cartilage roof line (1 = correct, 2 = incorrect) (**b**) An example of a correctly and an incorrectly drawn bony roof line (1 = correct, 2 = incorrect, fatty tissue and sinusoids at the lower limb were not excluded and the line is cutting through the bony echo instead of just touching it as described). (**c**) Correctly drawn measurement lines. The three lines do not necessarily intersect at a single point

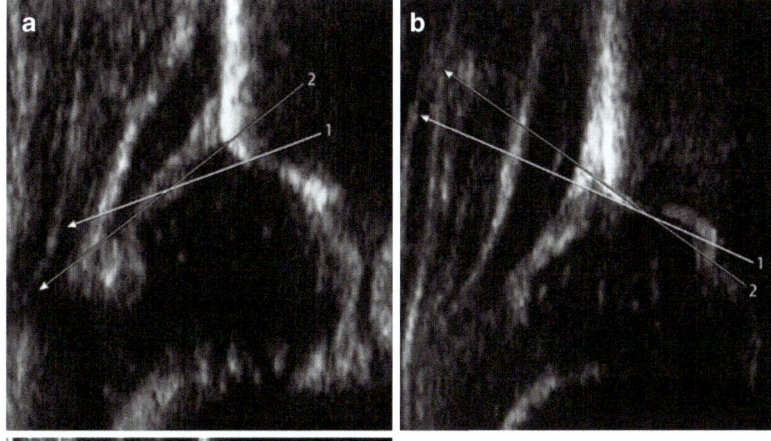

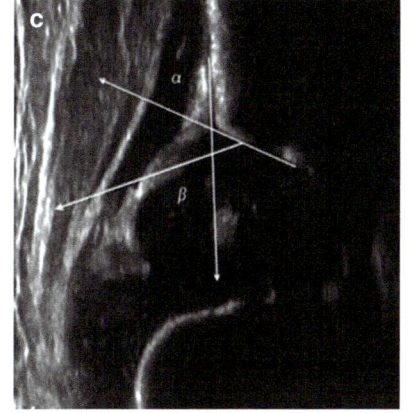

6.6   Summary

Conclusion
- Acetabular roof line:
  - Tangential from the lower limb just touching the bony socket (bony roof contact point is seldom the turning point).
  - Be careful of the echoes in the area of the lower limb: Sinusoids, fatty tissue, fovea centralis, possibly with ligament attachment.

- Baseline:
  - Drawn tangentially from the attachment of the proximal perichondrium, which is anatomically the rectus tendon attachment, to the ilium caudally (just touching the bone).
  - Baseline is not always parallel to the edge of the image.
- Cartilage roof line:
  - From the turning point through the centre of the labrum. Always search for the turning point from the bottom to the top (caudal to cranial), concavity–convexity.
- These three lines rarely intersect at one point.

References

1. Zieger M, Schultz D. Ultrasound of the infant hip. Part III: Clinical application Pediatr Radiol. 1987;17:226–32.

2. Graf R, Tschauner C, Schuler P. Ist die Hüftsonographie notwendig und unter welchen Voraussetzungen kann sie eingesetzt werden? Pädiat Prax. 1986;34:129–39.

3. Graf R. Sonographie der Säuglingshüfte. Ein Kompendium. 4th ed. Stuttgart: Enke; 1993.

Classification by Type of Sonograms of the Hip Joint

7.1 Basic Principles

In order to assess the status of a hip joint, it is necessary to classify the bony and cartilaginous coverage in relation to age: "What is normal at what age?"

Since the components of the hip joint—the femoral head and socket—influence each other, the femoral head leaves its mark during the dislocation process. These changes in the bone and cartilage roof can be classified using sonograms, giving a clear picture of the dislocation process. The level of the dislocated femoral head is not so important, but rather the pathology of the socket caused by the dislocation process.

The advantages of the upright image projection (erect right hip joint) have already been described (p. 21). The image description is subjective, but the method forces a systematic approach to the assessment of the hip joint and prompts the assessor to reduce the structures of the hip joint into three essential anatomical structures, ultimately leading to a preliminary diagnosis (classification) (Fig. 7.1).

A safety check is ensured through measurement: if there is a discrepancy between description and measurement, the examiner is forced to recheck both systems, has it been measured incorrectly or described incorrectly? Ultimately, the decision is verified by measurement.

The structures to be described are:

- bony roof of the acetabulum
- contour of the bony rim
- cartilaginous roof of the acetabulum

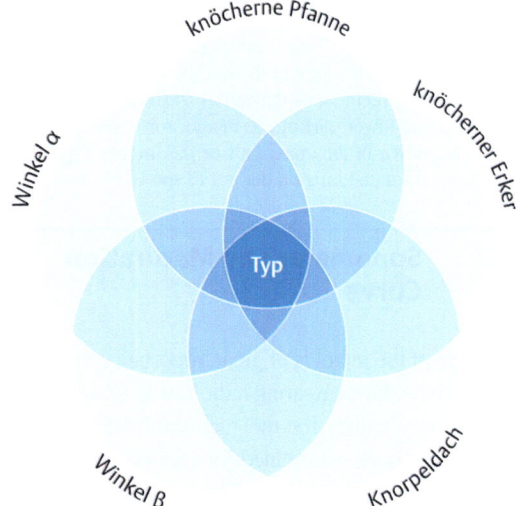

Fig. 7.1 Determination of the hip joint type. Narrowing down the type by considering as much information as possible in order to minimize errors

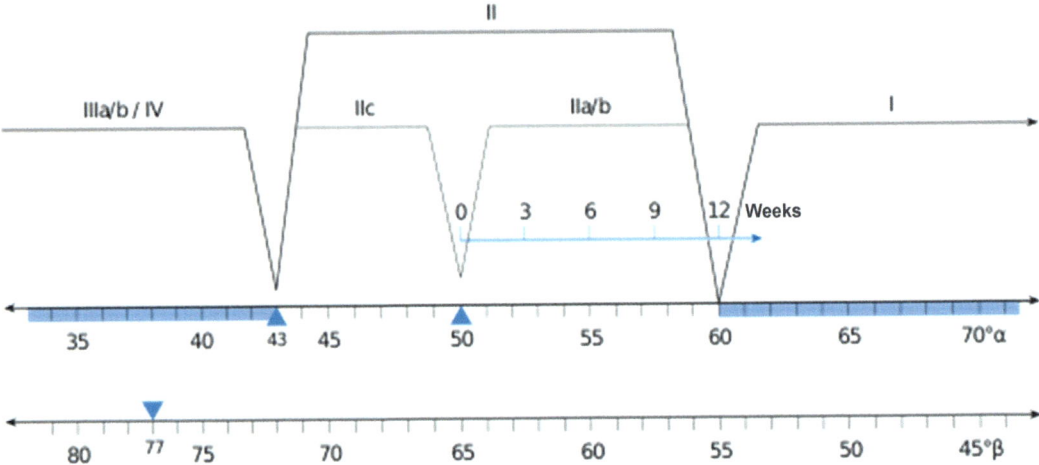

Fig. 7.2 Sonometer. Linear arrangement of the values of the α angle, black x-axis in the middle of the image, and opposing arrangement of the values of the β angle, black x-axis in the lower part of the image, for classifying hip types as shown in the upper half of the image: Type I on the right, disolated hips on the left (Type IIIa/b and Type IV), and Type II in the middle, subdivided into Type IIa, Type IIb, and Type IIc. Time scale for newborns (blue x-axis in the upper part of the image): for physiological hip maturation, the alpha angle should be at least 50° in newborns and at least 60° at 3 months of age

7.2   Sonometer and Maturation Curve

The age of the infant is of great importance in deciding the type. By comparing radiological findings and sonograms, values for the measurement angles α and β have been determined for various age groups. This has resulted in a graph, referred to as the "sonometer" (Fig. 7.2). Using this, the hip types can be determined for given α and β angles. The α angle in the sonograms and the AC angle in the X-ray have a certain relationship to each other [1, 2].

> **Note**
>
> α angle (sonography) + AC angle (X-ray) = 90°

Assuming a minimum level of enchondral ossification, the acetabular roof develops at birth to a minimum α angle of 50°, increasing to a minimum α angle of 60° by the third month of life due to the high potential for growth in the postpartum phase. Statistical studies showed that the mean α angle, not to be confused with the minimum value of 60, in Type I joints is 64.4° in the

third month of life [3, 4]. Assuming linear maturation (assuming the worst case so as to be on the safe side), the equation is calculated as follows:

The optimum α-angle at birth is 55°, not to be confused with the minimum maturity value of 50. The maturation curve (see Fig. 7.3) shows that the average natural maturation of untreated hip joints reaches 59° in the fourth week of life. Between the fourth and 16th week of life, the mean values as well as the standard deviation increase by only 4°. After the fourth month of life, a typical plateau pattern with angles between 64° and 65° is seen, which lasts until around the 11th month of life. By the 13th month of life, the mean α-value increase to 66°. The further maturation of the acetabular roof is described thereafter by the radiological AC angle by Tönnis.

> Note: Simplified for practical purposes: The hip matures very well in the first 5 weeks, and well until the end of the 12th week. After that, maturation potential slows down, the curve flattens. The minimum value for α angle at birth is 50°, at the end of the 12th week it is 60°.

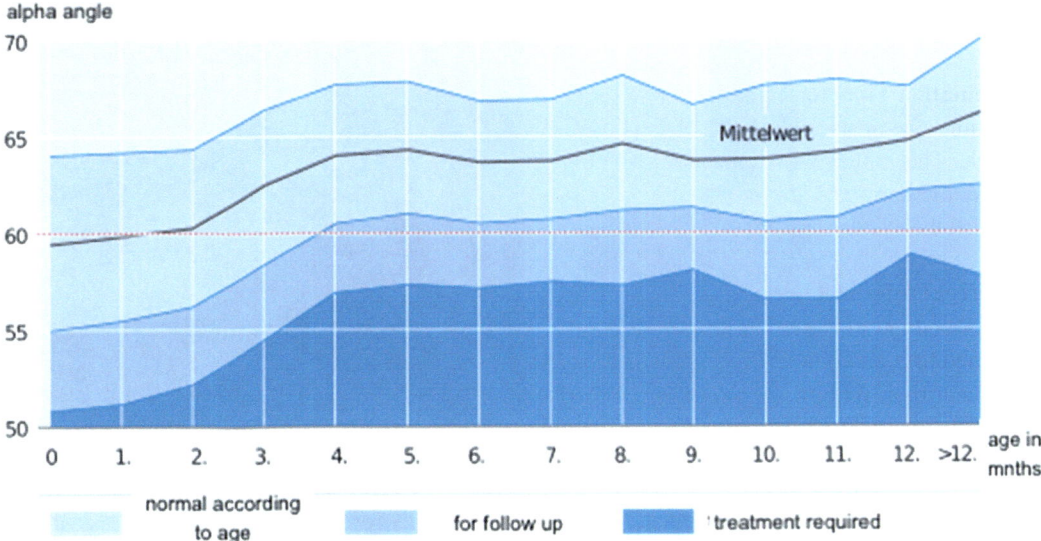

Fig. 7.3 Maturity curve. Values for the α angle in a longitudinal study in healthy infants. For values within the first standard deviation, babies have to be followed up and for values within the second standard deviation, treatment should be started

7.3   Sonographic Hip Types and Differentiation

7.3.1   Hip Types

Type I

Type I corresponds to a mature hip joint (Fig. 7.4). Mature means that at the end of the 12th week, the hip joint has reached a precisely defined level of ossification of the bony acetabulum. The bony roof is good, the bony rim area, or most lateral point of the acetabulum is usually blunt (see Fig. 7.4c), rarely angular (see Fig. 7.4b), and the cartilage roof covers the femoral head. The bony roof angle α, measures 60° or more. Type I can be present in newborns, but Type I should be reached at the latest by the end of the third month of life (Fig. 7.5).

Another subdivision can be made by measuring the cartilage roof angle β:

- Type Ia: β angle less than 55°, the cartilaginous roof extends widely over the femoral head
- Type Ib: β angle greater than 55°, relatively short cartilaginous roof

The distinction between Type Ia and Type Ib does not currently have any practical significance. It is a variation of a normal, mature hip (comparable to having blond or black hair). Possibly the cartilaginous roof may continue to develop differently until the end of growth, and a potential significance in regards to arthritic changes may be shown in future research studies [5]. Hypothesis: shallower acetabulum (Type Ib?) could be more prone to labral degeneration and tears, while deep acetabulum (Type Ia?) could be more prone to impingement syndromes.

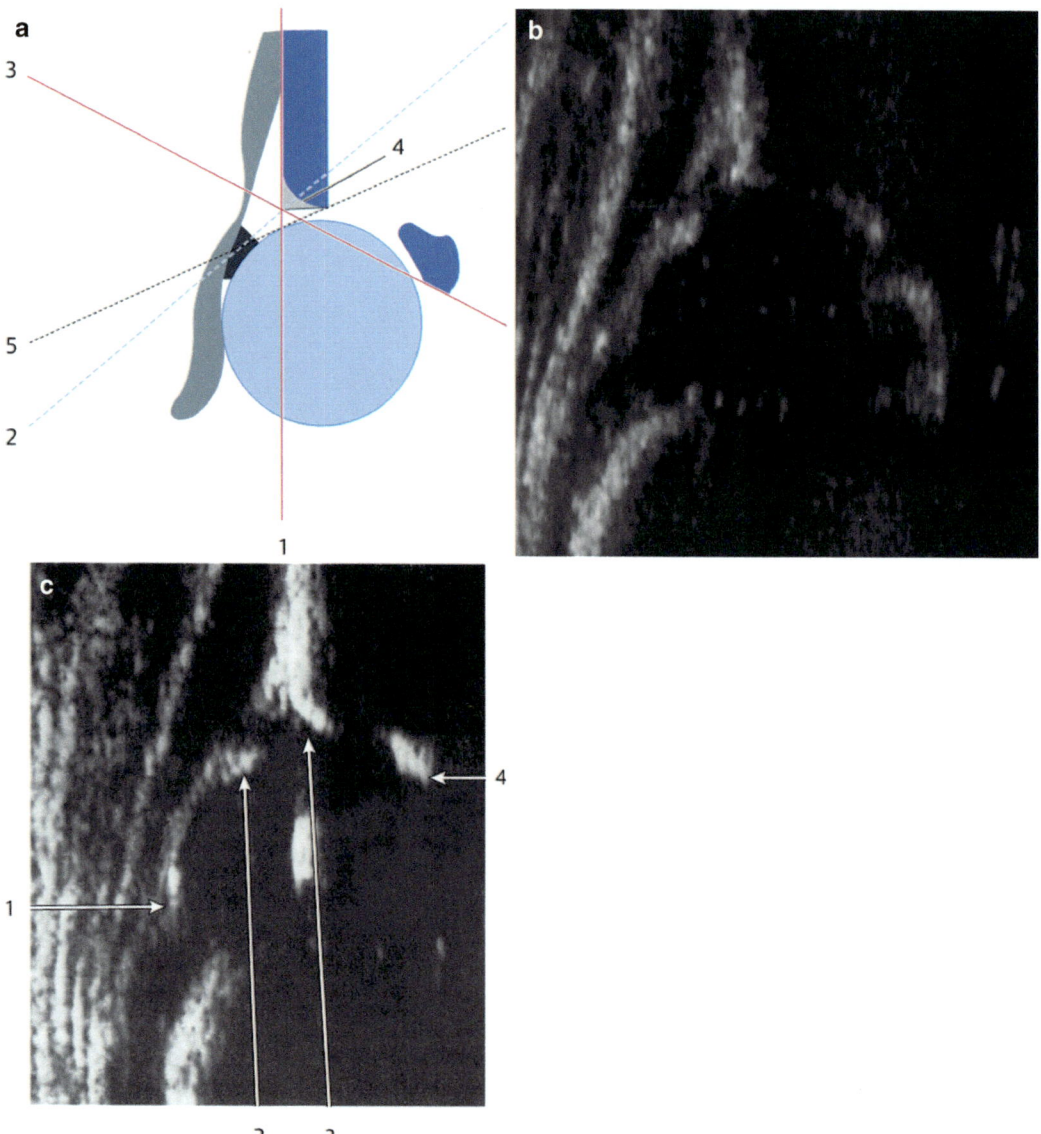

Fig. 7.4 Type I hip joint (**a**) Schematic drawing of a Type I hip joint with an angular (can also be described as sharp) and blunt bony rim (1 = base line, 2 = cartilage roof line with angular bony rim, 3 = bony roof line with angular bony rim, 4 = blunt bony rim, 5 = cartilage roof line with blunt bony rim) (**b**) type I with angular bony rim (**c**) type I with blunt bony rim (1 = synovial fold, 2 = labrum, 3 = blunt bony rim, 4 = lower limb of the ilium)

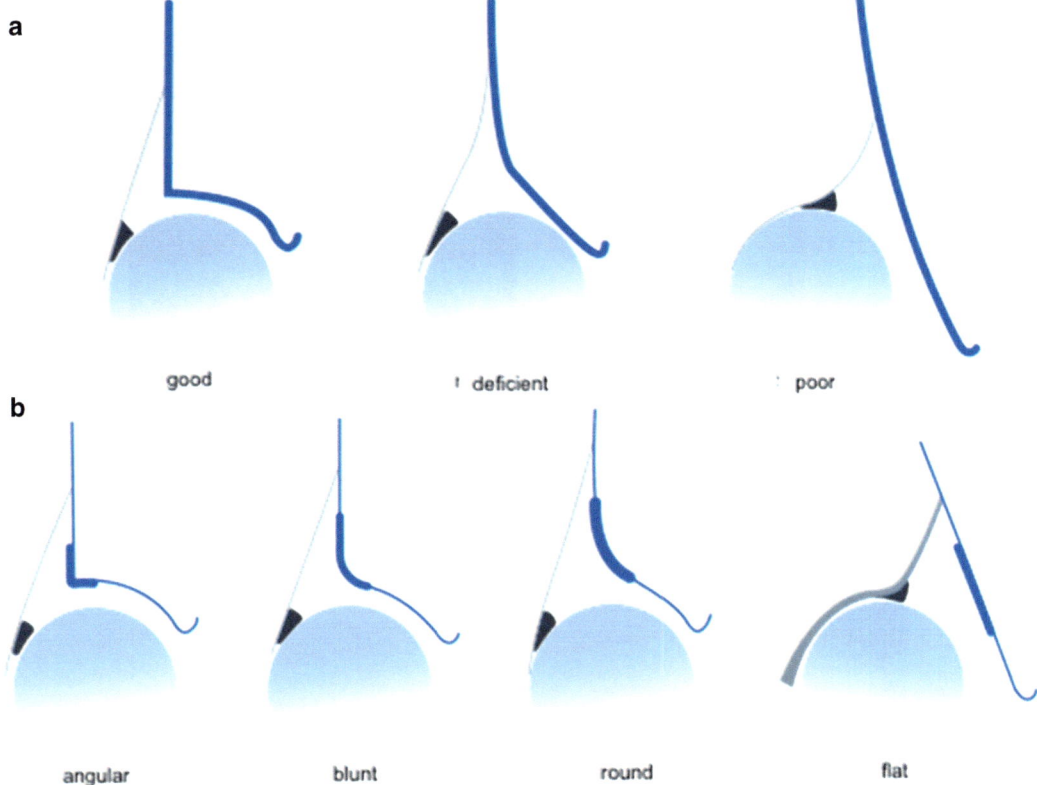

a

good   ᵗ deficient   ᵗ poor

b

angular   blunt   round   flat

Fig. 7.5 Schematic representation Type I-III (**a**) various shapes of the bony socket (**b**) description of the bony rim as either angular or blunt: Type I, round: Type II, flat: Type III

Type II

This type includes hip joints with various degrees of physiological and pathological delays in the ossification process of the acetabulum (Fig. 7.6). Subdivision depends on the age of the infant, younger or older than 12 weeks, and the extent of delay of the ossification process.

Type IIa

Type IIa occurs when the α-angle is between 50 and 59° in children younger than 12 weeks. This hip type corresponds to a physiologically immature hip joint. Such joints may initially appear dysplastic, but they are acceptable for their age:

They are immature, but not pathological (Fig. 7.7).

Type IIa hips can be further divided into Type IIa + and Type IIa- [6]. This division allows for the estimation of the growth potential. By referring to the corresponding timeline on the sonometer, one can determine the minimum alpha angle that should be reached in each week of life. This way, early onset of delayed maturation can be identified:

- Type IIa- hips are hip joints that already show a maturation deficit and are thus lagging behind in the expected alpha angle according to the age.

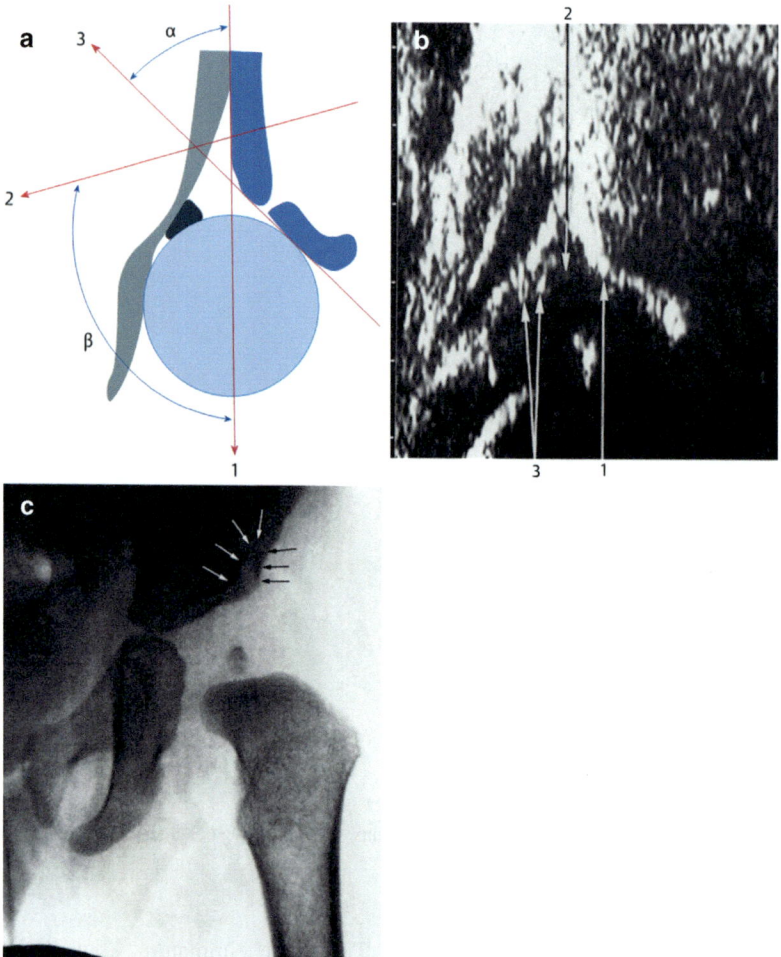

Fig. 7.6 Type II hip joint. Note: The images b and c are historical pictures from the year 1981. (**a**) Schematic drawing of a right Type II hip. The bony roof is deficient, with a round bony rim and the cartilage roof is covering the femoral head (α = bony roof angle, β = cartilage roof angle, 1 = baseline, 2 = cartilage roof line, 3 = bony roof line) (**b**) Left hip joint, at 9 months. The bony rim is round, with a deficient bony roof. The cartilage roof is covering, so it is a Type II hip joint. The plane passes through the bony rim defect corresponding to the X-ray image in **c** (1 = bony rim, 2 = the plane goes through the bony rim defect, 3 = labrum (**c**) Left hip dysplasia. Bony rim defect marked with arrows between the anterior and posterior part of the acetabular roof (corresponds to **b**, No. 2)

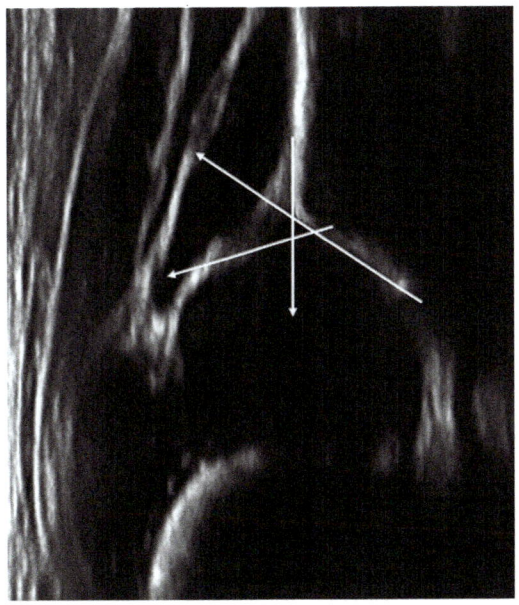

Fig. 7.7 Type IIa hip joint. Example of a Type IIa joint in a 4-week-old baby. The bony roof is adequate, the bony rim is round, and the cartilaginous roof covers the femoral head. The α angle measures 58°, and the β angle measures 78°. The joint has reached more than the minimum maturity level for that age, hence Type IIa+

- Type IIa + joints have reached the minimum stage of maturation expected according to age, or have exceeded it.

Practical tip
After the third newborn examination in Germany, where the general hip ultrasound screening takes place, was moved forward to the 4th–5th week of life, the following new recommendation for the management of infant hips in Type IIa + and Type IIa- is as follows:

- Hip joint at 4 weeks old:
- α angle between 52 and 59° (Type IIa+): follow-up recommended
- α angle = 50 or 51° (Type IIa-): in need of treatment
- Hip joint at 6 weeks old:
- α angle between 55 and 59° (Type IIa+): follow-up recommended
- α angle less than 55° (Type IIa-): in need of treatment

Type IIb
The α-angle in this type also falls between 50 and 59°, but in an infant that is older than 12 weeks. At this age, this hip joint corresponds to a dysplastic joint. The bony socket is deficient, the bony rim is round, but the cartilage roof still covers the femoral head (Fig. 7.8). If the bony rim appears angular instead of round, this indicates ossification and is considered to have a favourable prognosis.

Caution
Type IIa and Type IIb only differ in terms of age: bony coverage that is acceptable for a hip at age 4 weeks, is insufficient at age 4 months.

Type IIc
Type IIc corresponds to a critical hip ("Critical Range") or a hip in the danger zone with risk of dislocation = severe dysplasia, regardless of age (Fig. 7.9). The shape is highly dysplastic, the

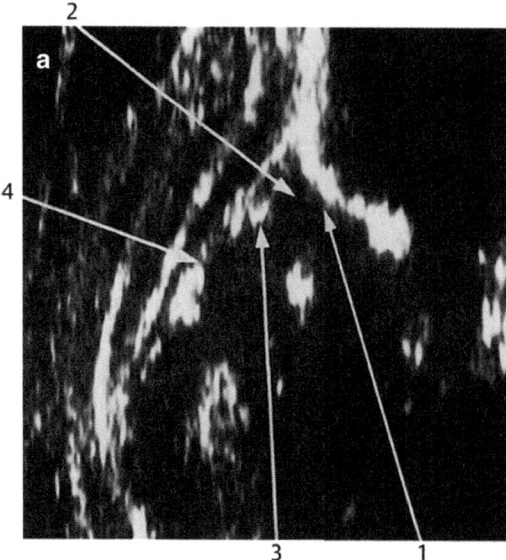

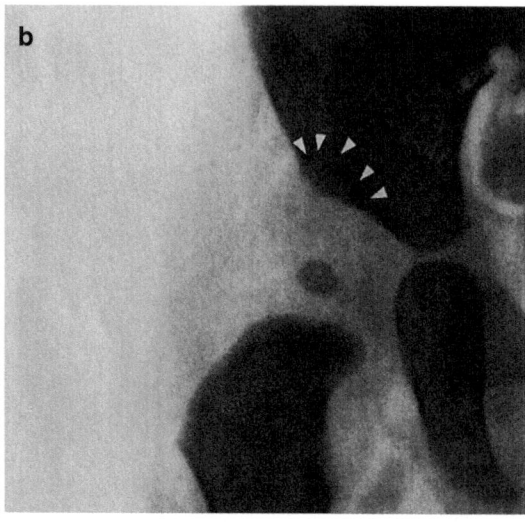

Fig. 7.8 Type IIb hip joint (**a**) Three-month-old baby. The bony roof is deficient, the bony rim is round, and the cartilaginous roof covers the femoral head. Note: The image is from 1987 with the precision standards of that time (1 = bony rim, 2 = cartilage roof, 3 = labrum, 4 = joint capsule) (**b**) X-ray corresponding to **a**. There is a severe bony rim defect. Only the posterior part of the acetabular roof is well developed. The bony rim defect is marked with arrows

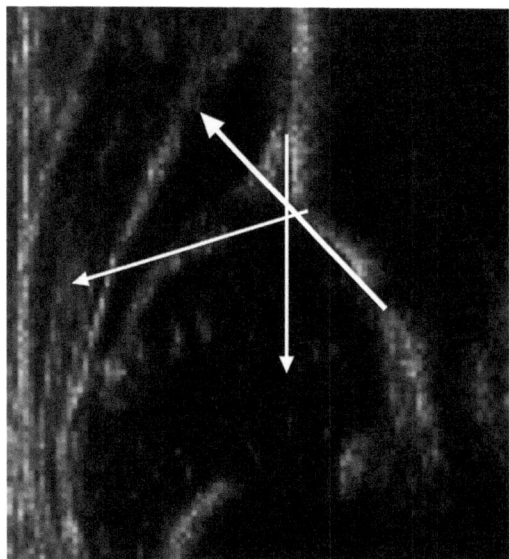

Fig. 7.9 Type IIc hip joint. Newborn hip joint. The bony roof is severely deficient, the bony rim is round to flat, and the cartilage roof is still covering. The α angle is 44°, and the β angle is 75°. Therefore, it is classified as Type IIc hip

bony rim is round to flat, and the cartilage roof still covers the femoral head. The α-angle measures 43–49° (Type IIc range), and the cartilage roof angle β is smaller than 77°. It is essential to measure both angles to differentiate it from a Type D hip (decentered hip).

Type D

In this type, the hip joint is starting to become decentred (Fig. 7.10). The α-angle is 43–49°, same as with a Type IIc hip, but the β-angle is greater than 77°. The Type D hip is the first stage of a decentring hip joint. It cannot be referred to as "Type IId" because all Type II joints are centred hip joints, while a Type D hip is the first stage of a decentred joint. Therefore, Type D hips are inherently unstable and do not need to undergo additional stress testing (p. 98).

Fig. 7.10 Type D hip joint (**a**) Four-week-old baby. The bony roof is severely deficient, the bony rim is round to flat, and the cartilaginous roof is displaced. The α angle measures 46°, and the β angle measures 90°. Therefore, it is classified as a Type D hip. (**b**) X-ray image corresponding to (**a**), with beginning subluxation (**c**) Differentiation between Type IIc and Type D using a sonometer. The α angle falls within the Type IIc range for both types. If the β angle is less than 77°, it is a Type IIc; if it is greater than or equal to 77°, it is a Type D hip joint

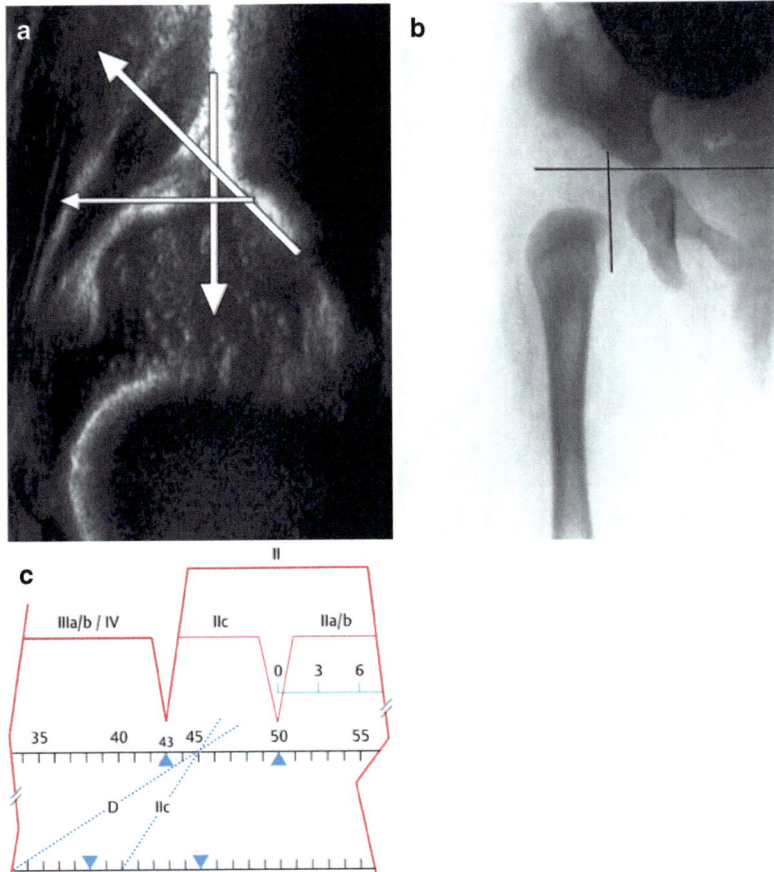

Practical tip

Stress test measurement of instability.

If a Type IIc hip can be converted into a Type D hip by a sonographic stress test, with the cartilage roof being displaced cranially under pressure and the β angle becoming greater than 77°under stress, this hip is referred to as "type IIc unstable". If the β angle remains less than 77° under stress, it is referred to as "type IIc stable".

Type III

Due to caudo-cranial shear forces on a poor bony roof, the cartilaginous roof of the acetabulum is deformed in a typical way by the femoral head, which is dislocating cranially. The femoral head is decentred in Type III. The majority of the cartilage roof is displaced cranially, while a smaller portion is pressed caudally towards the original acetabulum. The cartilage portion pressed downwards separates the original acetabulum from the secondary acetabulum that is created by the pressure of the dislocating femoral head and was called the "neolimbus" by Ortolani.

Type IIIa

In this type, there are no structural abnormalities in the cartilage of the acetabular roof. The typical sonographically echo-free hyaline cartilage of the acetabular roof is present (Fig. 7.11).

Type IIIb

In Type IIIb, structural disturbances of the cartilage are evident, resulting in altered echogenicity of the cartilage roof (see Fig. 7.12). The causes are the pressure and shear forces exerted

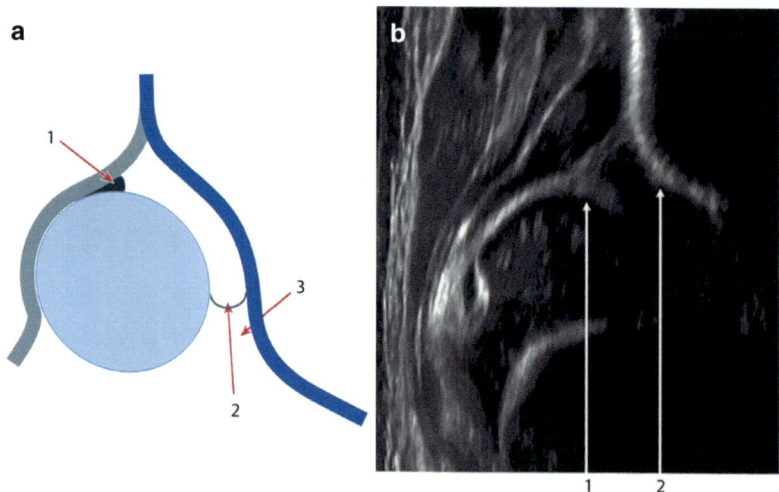

Fig. 7.11 Type IIIa hip joint (**a**) Schematic drawing of the right hip. Dislocation, Type III (1 = labrum, 2 = caudally compressed cartilage roof, 3 = acetabulum) (**b**) Eight-week-old hip joint. The bony roof is poor, the bony rim is flat, and the cartilaginous roof is displaced cranially and is hypoechoic. The findings correspond to a Type IIIa hip. Caution: The lower limb of the ilium can no longer be clearly visualized as the femoral head has already left the standard plane (1 = labrum, 2 = bony rim)

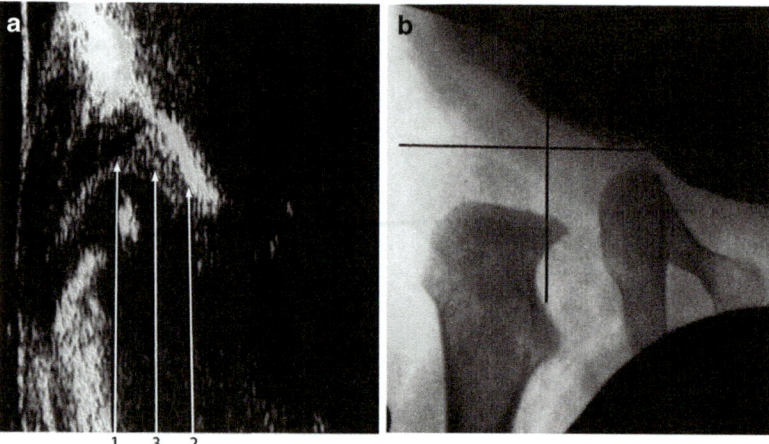

Fig. 7.12 Type IIIb hip joint (**a**) Sonogram of the right hip, 6 months old baby, showing significant echogenicity of the cartilaginous roof. The bony roof is poor, the bony rim is flat, the cartilaginous roof is echogenic and displaced cranially. The lower limb of the ilium is outside the standard plane and is not visible. Note: The sonogram is from the year 1985! (1 = labrum, 2 = bony rim, 3 = cartilaginous roof) (**b**) X-ray image of (**a**): Diagnosis of grade 2 dislocation according to Tönnis

by the dislocated femoral head on the hyaline cartilage roof, ultimately leading to fibrocartilaginous degeneration of the displaced acetabular roof cartilage (see Fig. 3.43). Due to early screening, Type IIIb hips have almost disappeared.

Mildly dislocated Type III joints can sometimes still be visualized in the standard plane. In these cases, they can also be measured: the α angle is less than 43°. If the dislocation is of a higher degree, the femoral head usually exits the standard plane, and these joints can no longer be measured. However, they can still be assessed, as the diagnosis is made morphologically based on the direction of displacement of the cartilaginous roof (differentiation between Type III and Type IV).

> **Learning point**
> The special morphological characteristic of Type III joints is that the majority of the cartilaginous roof is displaced cranially, causing the perichondrium to be pushed cranially as well.

Type IV

In Type IV hips, the femoral head is decentred. The entire cartilaginous roof is pressed in a medio-caudal direction towards the true acetabulum (Fig. 7.13). No cartilage roof is visible above the femoral head. This means that the displaced cartilage significantly hinders the reduction of the femoral head into the acetabulum. The prog-

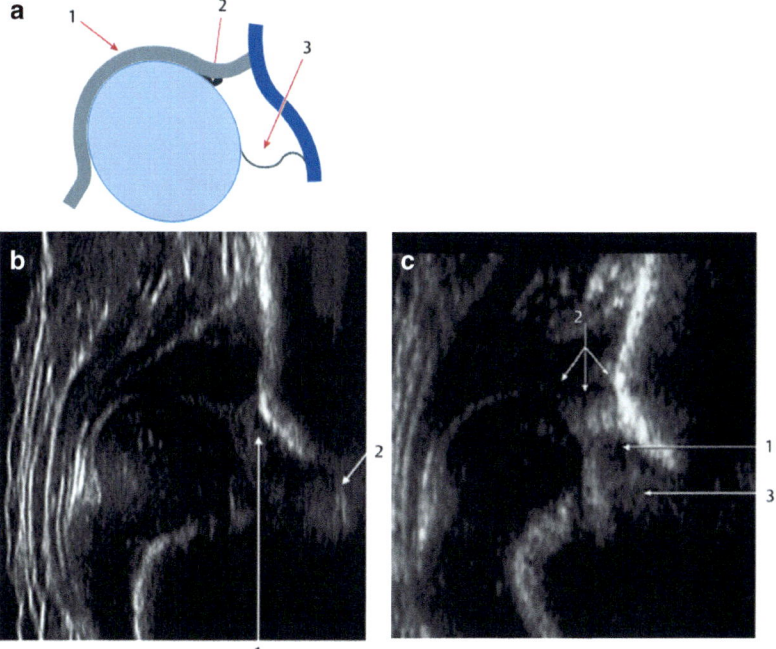

Fig. 7.13 Type IV hip joint (**a**) Schematic picture. The femoral head presses the hyaline cartilage together with the labrum downwards, towards the true socket. The structures are compressed between the femoral head and the bony socket (1 = joint capsule, 2 = labrum, 3 = caudally compressed cartilaginous roof) (**b**) Four-week-old hip joint Type IV. The femoral head is decentred, more laterally than cranially. The cartilaginous roof is compressed between the femoral head and the bony roof. There is no cartilaginous roof cranial to the femoral head and the proximal perichondrium is horizontal. Increased echoes in the depth of the acetabular fossa as a sign of increased fatty tissue (pulvinar) (1 = compressed cartilaginous roof, 2 = pulvinar in the depth of the acetabular fossa) (**c**) Hip Type IV. The femoral head compresses the acetabular roof cartilage between it and the iliac bone. The proximal perichondrium is horizontal or goes downwards. The depth of the acetabular fossa is filled with fatty tissue (1 = compressed cartilaginous roof, 2 = proximal perichondrium, 3 = pulvinar in the depth of the acetabular fossa)

nosis of a Type IV joint is significantly worse than that of a Type III joint.

Differentiation Type III/Type IV joints
The labrum is never "inverted", only the base of the labrum is pushed downward. It is never the obstacle to reduction. The obstacle to reduction is the acetabular roof cartilage, which is pressed more (Type IV) or less (Type III) downwards.

Type III and Type IV joints are, according to definition, decentred joints. The term subluxation (similar to "a little bit pregnant") is a clinical term and not a reflection of patho-anatomy; therefore, it should not be used in the sonographic classification.

Practical tip
Methodically, Type III and Type IV joints can be differentiated by considering the direction of the proximal perichondrium (Fig. 7.14): since the cartilage roof is hypoechoic or echo-free, it can only be delineated by the surrounding structures. The perichondrium is fixed to the cartilage roof and is the indicator of where the hyaline cartilaginous roof is located—cranial or caudal? The position of the labrum is irrelevant in this case. If the perichondrium

extends cranially, there must still be cartilage above the femoral head, indicating a Type III joint. If it extends horizontally to the bony acetabulum or in a cup-shaped manner, going downwards before rising towards the bony acetabular roof, a Type IV joint is present.

7.3.2 Differentiation Between Structural Pathological Changes and Ossification

The physiological ossification of the socket can cause echoes similar to those of pathological structural changes. Ossification can be found in centred joints (see Fig. 7.15) and lead to an improved shape of the bony rim, whereas pathological structural changes only occur in decentred (Type III and Type IV) joints.

Learning point
- Secondary ossification: echogenic roof in centred hips.
- Pathological structural changes: echogenic roof in decentred hips.

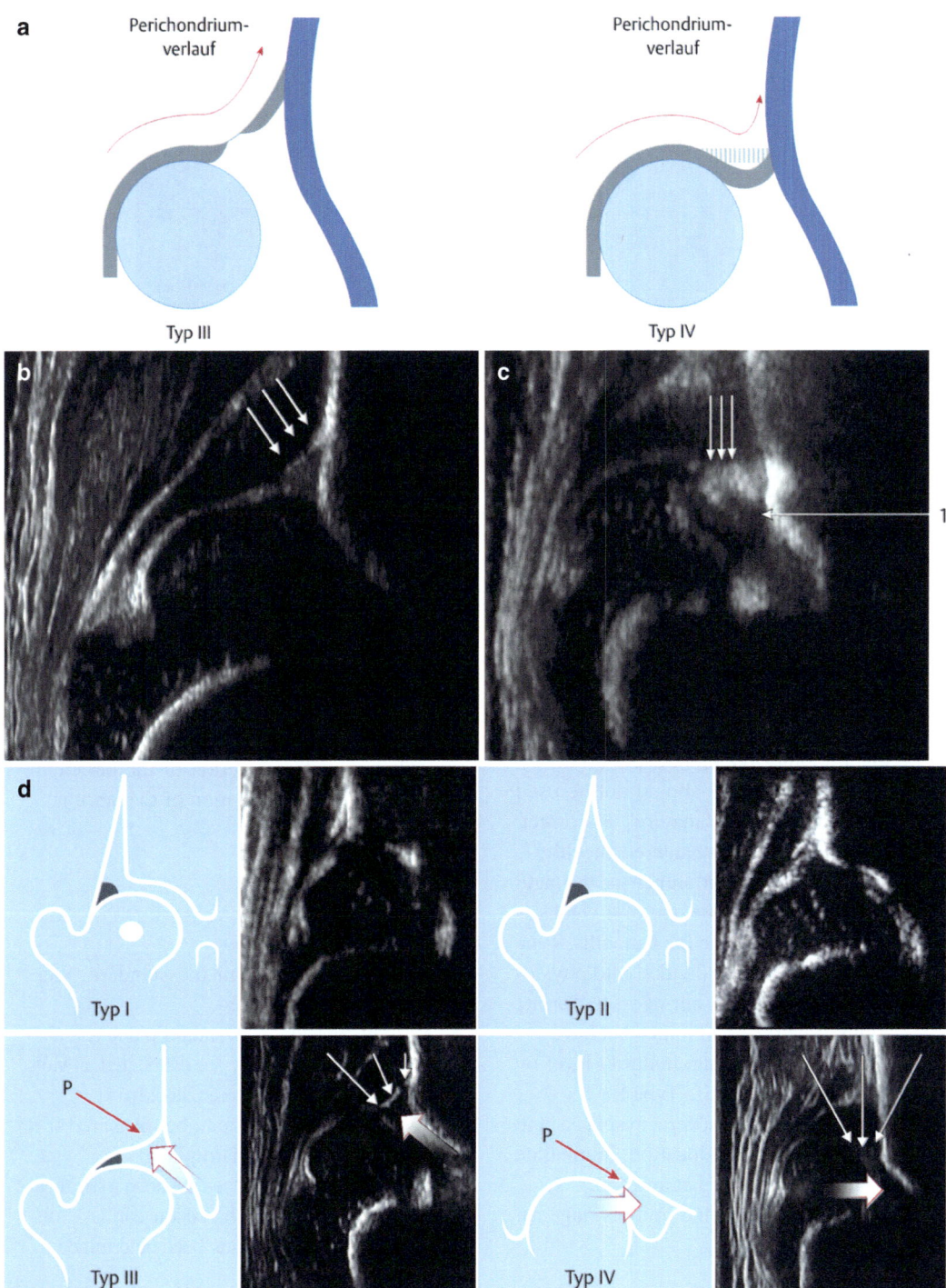

Fig. 7.14 Differentiation Between Type III and Type IV joints (**a**) Differentiation between Type III (**b**) and Type IV joints (**c**) based on the direction and course of the perichondrium and the cartilage roof (**b**) Differentiation between Type III (**b**) and Type IV joints (**c**): Hip Type III with cranially displaced cartilage roof, indirectly visible through the cranially directed proximal perichondrium (arrows) (**c**) Hip Type IV with caudally displaced cartilage roof and the proximal perichondrium going downwards (arrows) (1 = cartilaginous roof (**d**) Overview of the four hip types. The thick arrow marks the deformed cartilaginous roof. The thin arrows indicate the course of the perichondrium. P = perichondrium.

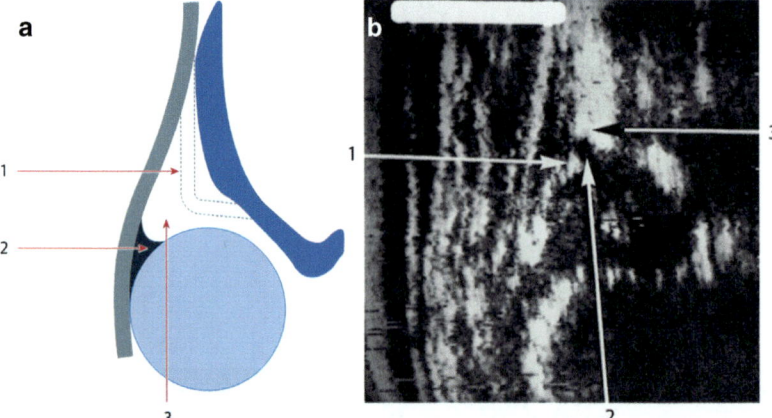

Fig. 7.15 Secondary ossification (**a**) schematic picture (1 = increasing sonographic echo from proximal to distal, 2 = labrum, 3 = not yet ossified cartilaginous roof) (**b**) Historical image from 1982. Mature hip joint Type I, well- developed angular bony rim extending over the cartilage roof (1 = labrum, 2 = largely ossified cartilaginous roof, 3 = os ilium with bony rim)

7.4   Summary and Conclusion

Types of hips
- Type Ia/b: These are variations of a mature joint (like blonde and brunette). The term "healthy" should not be used for Type I joints, "mature" is correct. Type IIa + is also considered "healthy".
- Type IIa/b: The difference is the age: what is normal at the age of 4 weeks is not enough coverage for 4 months. Type IIa hips are further divided into physiologically immature but age-appropriate joints Type IIa + and joints that have not reached the minimum maturity level by the third month of life Type IIa-.
- Type IIc: This is severe dysplasia and there is a risk of dislocation. Immediate treatment is required at any age.
- Type D: This is the initial stage of dislocation.

- Type III/IV: These types involve dislocated joints with differently deformed cartilaginous roofs, displaced cranially or caudally. The sonographic differentiation between Type III and Type IV is based on the direction of the perichondrium, not the position of the labrum.

Rules for measurement
- Only sonograms in the standard plane should be measured.
- Joints outside the standard plane can also be evaluated if they are dislocated, always use Checklist I before Checklist II.
- A dislocated joint can be measured if it is still in the standard plane.
- A dislocated joint does not need to be measured if the type, based on cartilage displacement has already been determined.

References

1. Melzer C. Röntgenbild—Sonographie—Anatomie (ein Vergleich). In: Schilt M, editor. Angeborene Hüftdysplasie und -luxation vom Neugeborenen bis zum Erwachsenen. Zürich: SGUMB-SVUPP-Eigenverlag; 1993. p. 69–77.
2. Melzer C. Korrelation Sono und Röntgen Orthopäde 1997; 26: 43–48.
3. Tschauner C, Klapsch W, Graf R. Das sonographische Neu- geborenenscreening des Hüftgelenkes—Luxus oder Notwendigkeit? Monatsschr Kinderheilkd. 1990;138:429–33.
4. Tschauner C, Klapsch W, Baumgartner A et al. "Reifungskurve" des sonographischen Alpha-Winkels nach Graf unbehandelter Hüftgelenke im ersten Lebensjahr. Z Orthop 1994; 132: 502–504.
5. Graf R. Sonographie der Säuglingshüfte. Ein Kompendium. 4th ed. Stuttgart: Enke; 1993.
6. Graf R. Hüftsonographie Grundsätze und aktuelle Aspekte Orthopäde 1997; 26: 14–24.

Evaluation of Hip Sonograms

8

There are clear guidelines for the evaluation of hip sonograms. The evaluation of many different data points and facts narrows down the diagnosis, making the classification by type safer and more reliable. Certain types are first excluded based on the age of the baby. Inconsistencies must not be accepted but should be clarified. A description of "cranially displaced acetabular roof" with an α-angle of 62° is inconsistent and must lead to a re-evaluation of the sonogram.

To avoid or minimize errors, the sequence of the different evaluation steps is important and must be strictly followed.

8.1 Documentation of Name, Date of Birth, Affected Joint, and Patient's Age

The age should always be known before the evaluation. It automatically narrows down the possible potential hip types. A 4-month-old joint cannot be classified as Type IIa.

8.2 Checklist I

(Anatomical Identification)
Anatomical identification must always be done before the usability check. This is to avoid classifaction of an incorrect hip sonogram, with misinterpretation of the anatomical echoes, when it is in fact not suitable for evaluation. If any point on Checklist I cannot be identified, the sonogram must not be used for diagnosis.

8.3 Checklist II

(Usability Check)
Check whether all the landmarks are present in the correct order. Exception: if the anatomical identification shows that it is a decentred joint, the lower limb of the ilium may be missing and a posterior plane may be present.

8.4 Description and Reporting

The report includes the morphological description of the bony and cartilaginous components of the acetabular roof using standard terms. Although it is largely subjective, it forces an analytical approach and narrows down the possible types. The description leads to a preliminary classification, which is confirmed by measurement. In Type I hips and especially in Type Ib joints, the bony rim is not always angular. Instead, the bony rim is often described as slightly rounded off. This type of bony rim is called blunt. Blunt bony rims are much more common than angular ones (Fig. Fig. 8.1).

An overview of the types with angles and descriptions, as well as the exception for Type II, can be found in Table. 8.1. When the terms in Table. 8.1 are used as in the horizontal row, they

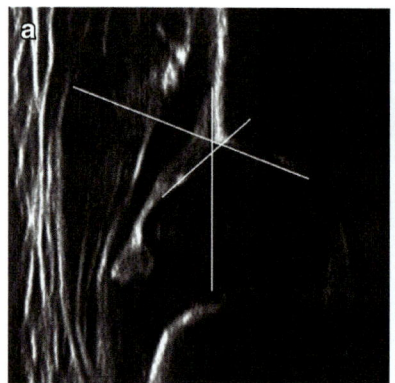
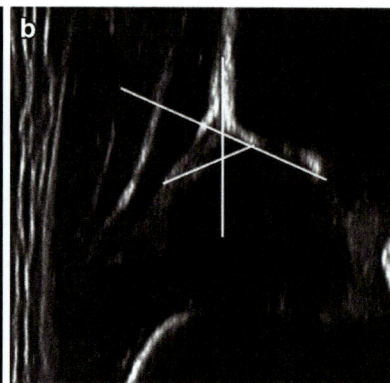

Fig. 8.1 Bony rim morphology (**a**) Five-week-old hip joint with good bone formation. The bony rim is angular, and the cartilaginous roof covers the femoral head. The α-angle measures 72°, and the β-angle measures 54°. This indicates a Type Ia joint. (**b**) Five-week-old hip joint. The bony roof morphology is good, but the bony rim is blunt, the cartilaginous roof covers the femoral head. The α-angle measures 66°, and the β-angle measures 63°. This is classified as a Type Ib joint

Table 8.1 description of hip types

Hip type	Description	Patient age	Bony coverage/α angle	Bony rim	Cartilage cover/β angle
I	Mature hip joint	Any age	Good α ≥ 60°	Angular/blunt	Covering Ia: β ≤ 55° Ib: β ≥ 55°
IIa	Physiological immature	< 12 weeks	Adequate, α = 50–59°	Round	Covering
IIa+	Physiologically immature according to age	< 12 weeks	Adequate, α ≥ age correlated angle on the sonometer	Round	Covering
IIa-	Physiologically immature with Maturation deficit	< 12 weeks	Deficient, α < age correlated angle on the sonometer	Round	Covering
IIb	Delayed ossification/ maturation	≥ 12 weeks	Deficient α = 50–59°	Round	Covering
IIc (stable/ Unstable	Critical joint Potential for dislocation	Any age	Severely deficient α = 43–49°	Round to flat	Still covering β < 77°
D	Joint in the process of dislocating	Any age	Severely deficient α = 43–49°	Round to flat	Displaced β ≥ 77°
IIIa/b	Decentred joint	Any age	Poor α < 43°	Flat	Cranially displaced IIIa: Without structural changes IIIb: With structural changes
IV	Decentred joint	Any age	Poor	Flat	Caudally displaced
Exception: Type II with bony remodelling	–	–	Deficient or adequate	Angular (secondary ossification due to remodelling)	Covering

The term covering cartilage roof (keeps the femoral head contained), applies exclusively to centred hips; the term displaced cartilage roof corresponds to a dislocated joint are correct and consistent. Therefore, the corresponding row in the description should, in general not be deviated from. The only exception is for Type II joints with further ossification: due to ossification around the bony rim, the bony rim may already be "angular" instead of "rounded." This can be considered prognostically favourable, as a sign of the beginning of development and improvement of the acetabular roof (the so-called remodelling).

8.5 Measurement Technique

Caution
If decentred joints are not in the standard plane, they can be given a type, based on whether the cartilage roof is pushed upwards or downwards, without being measured.

8.6 Determination of the Final Type

(Consistent Evaluation, Usability Check)
The description and the measurement must be consistent. Inconsistency between description and measurement should prompt a re-examination of the anatomical identification and a re-evaluation of the usability check. Since the description is subjective, the type is determined by measurement in borderline cases.

Practical tip
Estimation of coverage
 The description forces the examiner to deal with anatomical landmarks such as the bony rim, labrum and estimate the proportions of coverage, but a definite classification is not possible:

- If the bony socket covers more than "half" of the femoral head, it is probably Type I.
- If the bony socket covers less than "half" of the femoral head, there are two possibilities:

    - If the labrum is higher than the turning point, it is suspicious of a dislocation.
    - If the labrum is lower than the turning point, the hip joint is most likely still centred.

Learning point
Since the femoral head is not round, the centre of the head ("half") cannot be determined. Therefore, the provisional typing is only an estimate. All measurement methods that involve the diameter or centre of the femoral head in relation to the bony roof are therefore only eyeballing supported by numbers or percentages, and they lead to diagnostic errors.

8.7 Therapeutic Consequences

It must be decided if the infant can be discharged, followed up or if treatment is required.

Dynamic Stress Test

Hip ultrasound is fundamentally a dynamic examination: out of the many possible tomogram-like sections, dynamic, only one standard section, static, is selected to ensure reproducibility independent of the examiner. When pressure is applied to the femur in a cranial direction, as well as with rotational movements alone, there can be movement and displacement of the non-ossified cartilage roof. The following questions are undoubtedly significant:

- to what extent is this back-and-forth movement of the hip joint in the socket with subsequent deformation of the cartilage roof acceptable and within the normal range (elastic whipping).
- and at what stage are these movements pathological and thus damaging to the hip joint (true instability).

9.1 Clinical Instability and Sonographic Instability

Clinical instability refers to the relative movements of the femoral head in the hip joint and beyond the edge of the acetabulum with various examination manoeuvres such as Ortolani's sign, Barlow's sign, and dislocation and relocation movements. Extensive literature exists on various manual examination techniques. It is agreed that the reproducibility of the different sliding and snapping phenomena, as well as signs of instability, depend greatly on the examination technique and the skill and experience of the examiner. There are significant limitations to reproducibility. After all, 52.5% of pathological neonatal hips do not have risk factors or clinical signs. Additionally, clinically stable but dysplastic hips in the pre-dislocation stage, Type IIc, cannot be detected.

"Sonographic instability" refers to the observed movement of the femoral head out of the acetabulum with subsequent deformity of the cartilaginous roof, which can be quantified through measurement. Sonographic instability can, if necessary, thus be quantified and demonstrated independent of the examiner's skill and sense of touch.

9.2 Conducting the Stress Test

The sonographic stress test is performed in a similar manner to the clinical examination, except with the child in a lateral instead of supine position. After usual positioning, the ultrasound probe is placed correctly over the hip joint. Care should be taken to ensure that both hands of the examiner are supported on the bolsters of the cradle (Fig. 9.1). After finding the standard plane, the ultrasound probe is held with the right hand, while the left hand reaches for the knee joint and applies axial pressure in a cranial direction.

R. Graf et al., *Sonography of the Infant's Hip*, https://doi.org/10.1007/978-3-031-71949-3_9

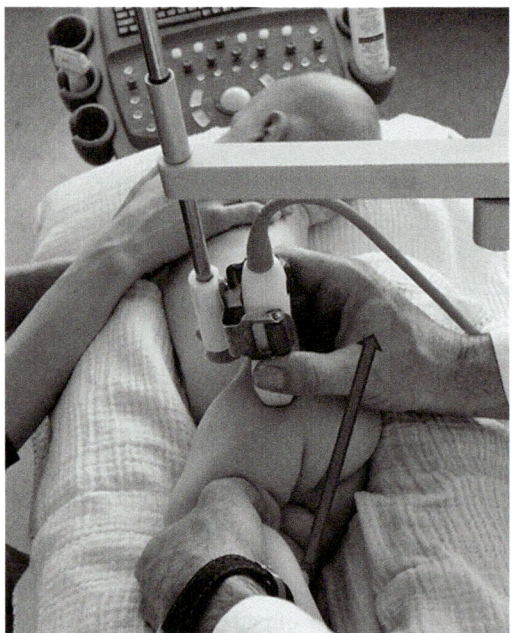

Fig. 9.1 Stress examination of the left hip. The right wrist rests on the bolster of the cradle to ensure secure guidance of the ultrasound probe and the ability to rotate the probe to adjust the plane. The left hand grasps the leg to be examined and can apply traction and pressure to the hip joint for the stress examination

Practical Tip

It is important that the right wrist is supported on the bolster of the cradle; otherwise, the standard plane can easily be lost. During the stress test, it is often necessary to readjust the ultrasound probe towards the decentring femoral head. This is easily achieved if the right wrist is supported.

A slightly adducted position of the hip joint makes the instability, if present, even more impressive. In sonographically unstable hips, the femoral head displaces proximally, taking the labrum with it (Fig. 9.2). When the pressure is taken off the femoral head, it slides back into its original position. In severely dysplastic hips, the upwards movement of the femoral head can be visualized sonographically just by the baby spontaneously flexing the hip.

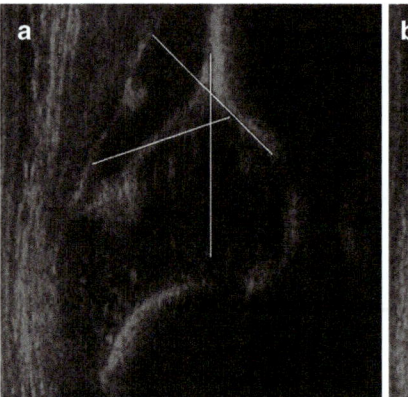
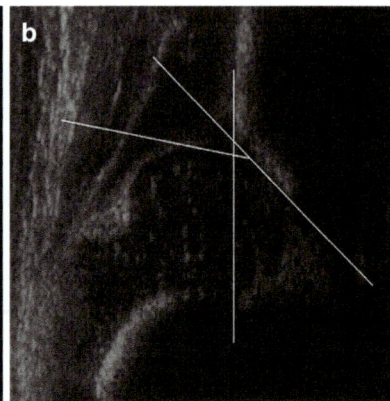
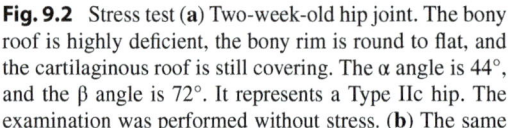

Fig. 9.2 Stress test (**a**) Two-week-old hip joint. The bony roof is highly deficient, the bony rim is round to flat, and the cartilaginous roof is still covering. The α angle is 44°, and the β angle is 72°. It represents a Type IIc hip. The examination was performed without stress. (**b**) The same hip joint as in (**a**), now with stress test. Under pressure, the femoral head moves significantly upwards. The α angle is still 44°, but the β angle is now 100°. The hip type now corresponds to a Type D based on the new sonographic measurement. Final classification: Type IIc—unstable

9.3   Elastic Whipping

Even in fully matured hips, a slight movement of the labrum, together with the cartilage roof can be observed when the proximal femur moves (Fig. 9.3). This is an adaptation process due to the physiological incongruities of the components forming the joint. Biomechanically and anatomically, the hip joint corresponds to a nut-shaped joint, not a ball-shaped joint. The type of the hip joint does not change with elastic whipping.

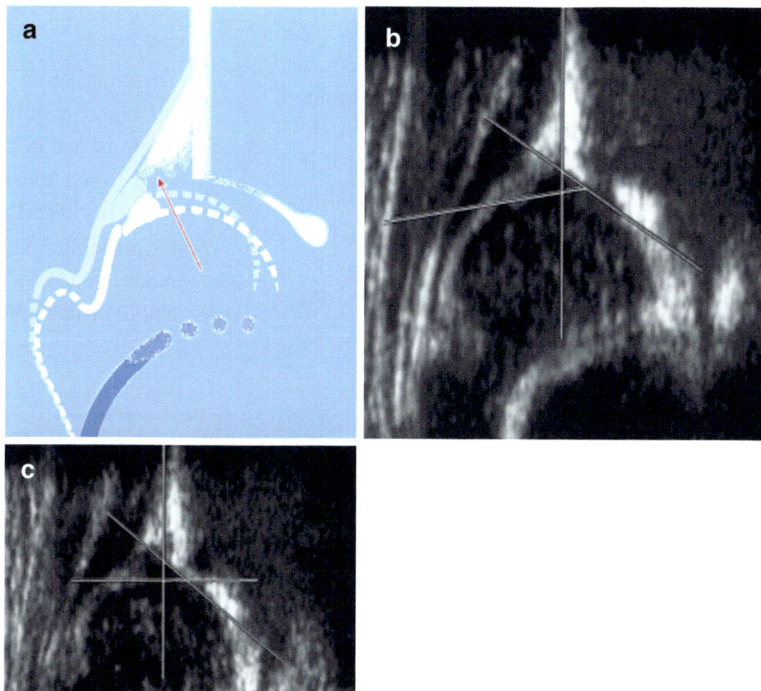

Fig. 9.3 Elastic whipping (**a**) Schematic picture. Even with good bony coverage, pressure, or rotation of the femoral head can displace the cartilaginous roof (arrow). This elastic whipping is not considered pathological as long as there is good bony coverage. (**b**) Example of elastic whipping. The α angle is 55° without stress, and the β angle is 74°. (**c**) Same hip joint as in (**b**), now under stress. With the same bony roof angle, the cartilaginous roof and labrum lift upwards (β angle = 89°): elastic whipping occurs

9.4 Typing of Sonographically Unstable Hip Joints

Naturally, decentred hip joints are inherently unstable (Type D, Type IIIa, Type IIIb, and Type IV). However, the important question to address is at what point does the harmless elastic whipping turn into pathological instability.

Learning point
A hip joint is sonographically unstable, when it is possible to change a Type IIc joint into a Type D hip under pressure. If this is the case, this hip joint is referred to as Type IIc unstable (see Fig. 9.2a and Fig. 9.2b). If a Type IIc cannot be converted into a Type D under pressure, this hip joint is referred to as Type IIc stable.

Through the distinction between Type IIc—stable and Type IIc—unstable, it is possible to diagnose instability objectively in borderline cases, independent of subjective clinical impressions.

Practical tip
The habit common in certain places of not drawing the cartilage roof line and not measuring the β-angle makes it impossible to classify Type IIc—stable, Type IIc—unstable, and Type D hips. This is a missed opportunity perpetuating the historic inability to differentiate pathological and therapeutically important instability from physiological movements (elastic whipping), irrespective of the experience and skill of the clinical examiner.

If the cartilage roof line is not drawn, the examiner is unable to provide documentary evidence of correctly identifying the essential structures of the labrum and turning point. In the case of misdiagnosis, this can cause legal problems.

Conclusion
- Elastic whipping: These are harmless movements of the hip joint and cartilage roof caused by capsular laxity or adaptations to physiological incongruities.
- Instability: This refers to pathological movements of the hip joint that cause damage to the acetabulum due to shearing forces.
- Differentiation between elastic whipping and instability: As long as the α angle is not in the Type IIc range, it is considered elastic whipping. If the α angle is in the Type IIc range, instability is possible. The exact distinction is made by classifying Type IIc as either stable or unstable.

9.5 Typing of Unstable Hip Joints

Learning point: The typing of the hip joint is generally done in a resting position, i.e. without "stress".

Sonographically unstable hips are either in the Type IIc range, or correspond to hip types D, III or IV. Of course, they can dislocate still further during the dynamic examination. For example, a Type III hip joint can transition into a Type IV hip when the femoral head is pushed cranially, and the cartilage roof slips completely below the femoral head. According to the definition, typing is done without stress; therefore, this hip joint would still be classified as Type III.

Further examples:

- A hip joint Type IIc is converted to a Type D by taking measurements during a stress test: in this case, the hip is Type IIc—unstable.
- A hip joint Type IIc is subjected to pressure, but it cannot be converted to a Type D when

measured. Therefore, it is a Type IIc—stable hip.

- An attempt is made to reduce a Type D hip. Under traction, it is successfully reduced, and in this position, the sonographic measurement would show a Type IIc. However, since hip joints are classified without stress, the diagnosis is Type D.

- A Type D hip is subjected to pressure. The hip joint deteriorates, the β-angle increases, but the α-angle remains within the Type IIc range. Therefore, it is a Type D hip.

Special Features and Sources of Errors

During the daily practice of hip ultrasound, typical, frequently recurring mistakes and special problems often arise. In the following section, the most common and important issues will be repeated summarized and supplemented with specific comments.

10.1 Questions of Nomenclature

Clarification of terminology:

- The term dislocation is a generic term and does not provide any details of the patho-anatomical deformities of the socket.
- The term subluxation at best means partially dislocated and does not have any patho-anatomical equivalent.

Therefore, the term subluxed can only be used in relation to a clinical examination.

- The term hip dysplasia refers to the malformation of the socket and is not related to age.

Since this term is no longer sufficient for a patho-anatomical assessment with corresponding consequences for treatment, the term "hip maturation disorder" is used for the varying degrees of defective ossification.

Depending on whether the femoral head is congruent with the socket or if this congruence is lost, we distinguish between centred and decentred joints:

- Decentred joints: Type D, Type IIIa, Type IIIb (nowadays very rare), and Type IV
- Centred joints: Type I, Type IIa, Type IIb, and Type IIc

In general, a Type II joint is described with a deficient or adequate bony roof, rounded bony rim, cartilaginous roof covering the femoral head. In cases of remodelling or delayed maturation, the first sign of acetabular ossification is the angular appearance of the bony rim. The description of a deficient or adequate bony roof, angular bony rim (exception), and cartilaginous roof covering the femoral head, indicates a Type II joint with further ossification of the cartilaginous roof.

The commonly used terms for the bony socket are either deficient or adequate and are used differently depending on what we want to describe:

- Deficient should be used in the sense of too little, not acceptable, not tolerable for Type-IIa- and Type-IIb joints.
- Adequate should be used in the sense of age-appropriate or acceptable for Type-IIa + joints (see Fig. 10.1).

R. Graf et al., *Sonography of the Infant's Hip*, https://doi.org/10.1007/978-3-031-71949-3_10

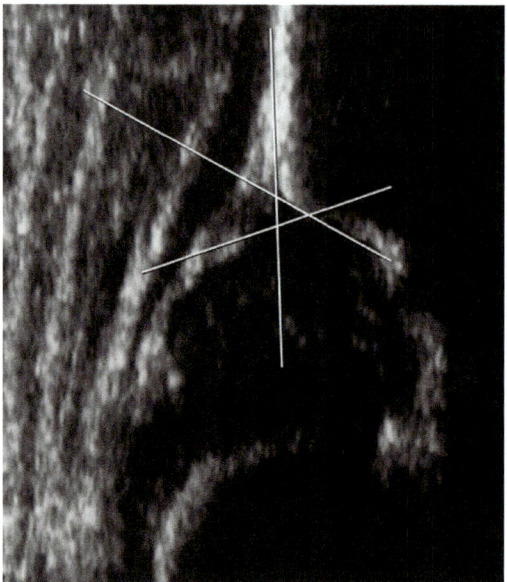

Fig. 10.1 Description of the bony roof. Six-week-old baby. The bony roof is adequate, the bony rim is round, and the cartilaginous roof covers the femoral head. The α angle is 58°, and the β angle is 75°. This is a hip type IIa+, which is acceptable

10.2 Most Common Errors in Practice

The most common errors encountered in daily practice will be mentioned again according to their importance. They will be discussed in the order of the methodical approach and their significance.

10.2.1 Errors during the Examination

Examination Time too Long
The time factor is often not taken seriously enough. The longer the examination, the more restless the baby and the more difficult it is to establish the standard plane.

Incorrect Order of Landmarks
The lower limb of the os ilium must always be identified first, and only then the mid plane of the acetabular roof. With the recommended scanning technique, the labrum is usually automatically visible at the same time.

Tilting Errors

> Learning point: Tilting mistakes must be strictly avoided

Tilting errors have enormous significance and can cause misdiagnosis (Fig. 10.2). They can lead to significant image distortion, especially with sector scanners, but also with obliquely positioned linear ultrasound probes or due to incorrect positioning of the baby. They can largely be avoided with the probe guide system.

Incorrect Positioning
Attention should be paid to the correct positioning of the infant. In addition to the cradle, an ultrasound probe guide system should be used.

10.2.2 Errors during the Anatomical Identification and the Usability Check

Incorrect Timing of Usability Check
The Checklist I must be performed on the sonogram before the usability check (Checklist II)—never the other way around. If the usability check is performed first, there is a risk of misinterpreting an echo in the depth of the acetabular fossa for the labrum, and incorrectly using a sonogram mistakenly thinking that all three landmarks are present, even if they are not.

Mistaken Identity
Classic errors of incorrect identification include not delineating the lower limb from the surrounding structures and the fovea centralis (see Fig. 10.3). Mistaking the labrum for the proximal perichondrium, which can be markedly compressed in decentred joints (see Fig. 10.4), or confusing it with the ischiofemoral ligament or the synovial fold.

> **Learning Point**
> Errors of anatomical identification are the primary cause of misdiagnosis.

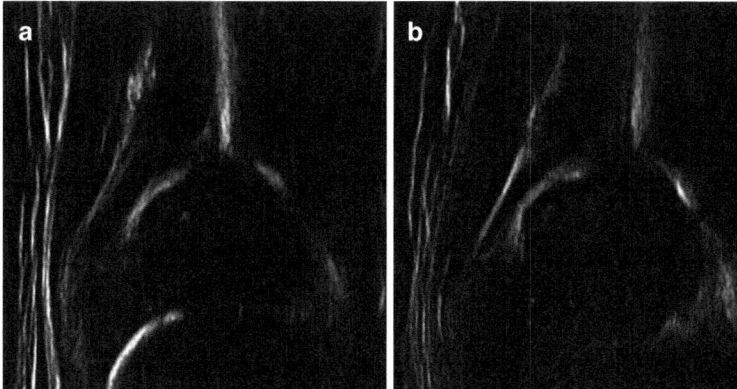

Fig. 10.2 Caudo-cranial tilting error (**a**) Correct sonogram. All anatomical echoes of checklists I and II are present: The three landmarks of checklist II are clearly visible, and the chondro-osseous border is also present, largely ruling out a caudo-cranial tilting mistake. There is no widening of the iliac silhouette or widening of the proximal perichondrium. Therefore, antero-posterior tilting errors are also excluded. (**b**) Same hip joint as in (**a**). Classical caudo-cranial tilting error leading to over-diagnosis. The femoral head appears elongated and oval, the bony socket can be described as poor, and the femoral head appears to be decentred. The tilting error can be recognized through the missing chondro-osseous border

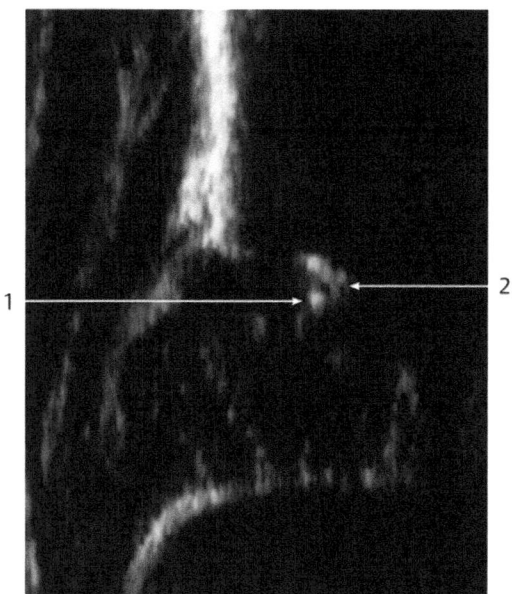

Fig. 10.3 Possibility of confusing the lower limb of the ilium with the central fovea (1 = central F with ligamentum teres, 2 = lower limb of the ilium)

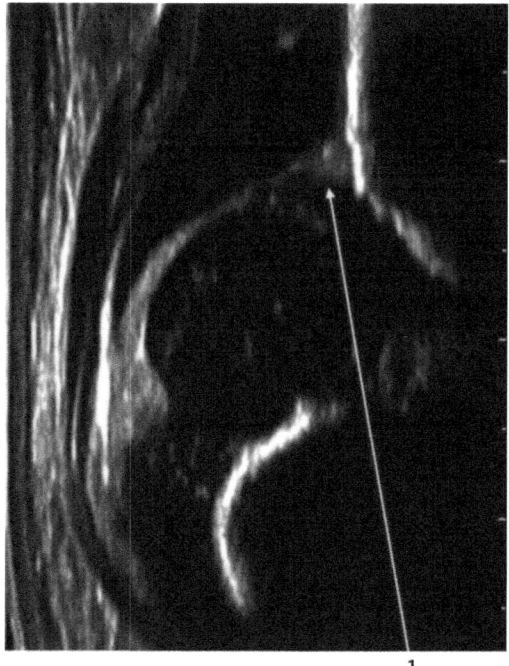

Fig. 10.4 Possibility of confusion between the labrum and the compressed proximal perichondrium (1 = perichondrium)

Errors in Distinguishing Type III/IV

The location of the deformed cartilage roof, not the labrum, is therapeutically and prognostically important. In order to determine the location of the deformed cartilage, the perichondrium which is attached to the cartilage, must be used to help identification:

- Type III: ascending proximal perichondrium
- Type IV: horizontal or cup-shaped direction of the proximal perichondrium

Incorrect Identification of the Turning Point

The turning point is the point of transition of the acetabular concavity to the convexity (counter-curvature). It is always to be sought from below (caudo-medially) to above (cranio-laterally) (Fig. 10.5) and is the most lateral point of the acoustic shadow. The turning point is rarely at the intersection of the baseline and bony roof line.

Incorrect Comparison Between Sonogram and X-Ray

There is a time lapse between the sonogram and the radiograph due to the different imaging modalities. Ossification can be detected 6–8 weeks earlier on the sonogram. Therefore, a

sonogram and a radiograph should never be compared on the same day. There is a correlation between sonographic α-angle and radiological AC value [1]:

10.3   Neglecting the Patient's Age

10.3.1 Age Limit for Hip Ultrasound

The use of sonography for the infant hip is limited by the ossification of the cartilaginous components of the hip joint. The limiting factor is the ossific nucleus of the femoral head, which can block the lower limb of the ilium by the acoustic shadow it creates. The limiting factor is therefore not age, but the degree of ossification of the femoral head.

10.3.2 Premature Infants

Premature infants have a higher proportion of immature joints, but not more joint pathology.

> **Beware**
> The hip joints of premature babies are classified according to their chronological age, but the treatment decisions are based on their gestational age.

For example, a 15-week-old infant with an α-angle of 58° and a β-angle of 72° is classified as Type IIb (delayed ossification). However, due to being born 6 weeks prematurely, the hip maturation age would be corrected to the ninth week of life. Therefore, the finding is "Type IIb, acceptable due to prematurity, recommended to be reassessed in 6 weeks".

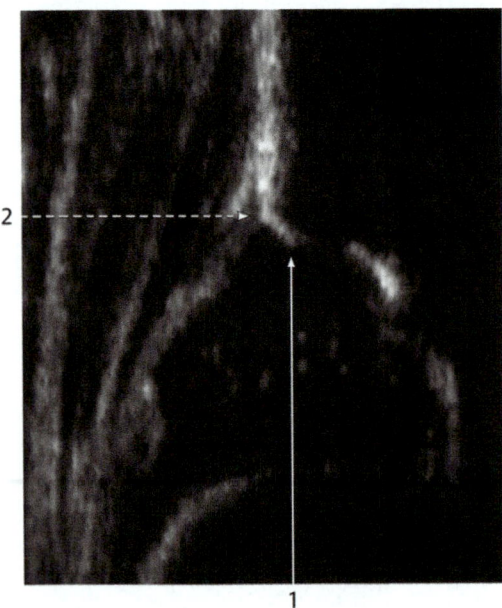

Fig. 10.5 Possible errors in determining the turning point. The correct definition of concavity to convexity leads to the correct identification of the turning point. If the turning point is sought in the wrong direction top to bottom instead of bottom to top, it would be sought too far proximal and therefore incorrectly identified (1 = correctly identified turning point, 2 = incorrectly identified turning point)

Reference

1. Melzer C. Korrelation Sono und Röntgen Orthopäde. 1997;26:43–8.

Ultrasound-Based Treatment

11

> **Remember**
> Result = diagnosis + treatment.

An early diagnosis is worthless unless it is acted upon with the appropriate immediate treatment. It is important to take the biomechanical situation into account when considering ultrasound-guided treatment.

The following explains the treatment algorithm based on the patho-biomechanical principles.

11.1 Maturation Curve

The maturation curve gives information about the growth and potential for ossification of the acetabular roof [1]. Essentially, this means that the hip joint has significant maturation potential in the first 6 weeks of life, which is still present in the second period from the sixth to the 12th week of life but decreases significantly by the 12th week of life. By the 16th week of life, it plateaus to a certain extent and changes only slightly. This behaviour is consistent with the clinical experience that even dislocated joints treated in the first 6-week period, have a very good chance of improving. In Type IIc hip joints, the healing rate can even be 100% [2, 3].

11.2 Basic Treatment Principles Based on Biomechanical Aspects

The starting point for any treatment has to be the analysis of the pathological anatomy of the hip joint, taking the maturation curve into consideration.

11.3 Treatment Goals

- Pathological anatomy should be corrected into the age-appropriate, normal anatomical structure of the hip joint.
- The ossification potential of the hip joint should be utilized in accordance with the maturation curve: a safe diagnosis should be made and, when necessary, treatment should start as soon as possible after birth.
- Damage to existing structures, especially to the growth areas of the acetabulum, and osteonecrosis of the hip should be avoided. Histological studies of the growth area of the acetabular roof [4] have confirmed how important early diagnosis is and have provided an explanation of what is a risk factor for hip dislocation.

R. Graf et al., *Sonography of the Infant's Hip*, https://doi.org/10.1007/978-3-031-71949-3_11

11.4   Stages of Treatment

The typing by sonography allows conclusions about the patho-biomechanical situation of the joint. Due to the process of dislocation of the femoral head, the acetabular roof has been mechanically deformed. Therefore, methods of treatment must be selected, that enable the forces in the hip joint to be redirected so that these deformities of the socket can be reversed to the normal morphology as appropriate for the age of the infant.

> **Learning point**
> Essentially, regardless of age, the hip joint has to go through an initial preparatory phase and then three further phases of treatment.
>   Starting from the worst-case scenario of a dislocated joint.
>
> - Reduction.
> - Retention.
> - Maturation.
>
>   Exception: see   newborn   screening (Sect. 11.5).

11.4.1 Preparation

Unfortunately, there may be unavoidable delays before treatment can be started, meaning that a dislocated hip cannot immediately be manually reduced or centred within the acetabulum using a temporary device. This usually happens in older children who already have significant restrictions of movement and adductor contractures [5]. In these cases, the hip joint needs to be prepared and surrounding soft tissue structures need to be stretched. Depending on the severity, this can be achieved through appropriate physiotherapy, or in severe cases, through extension treatment or an adductor tenotomy.

11.4.2 Reduction

Reduction of the femoral head is needed in cases of dislocated joints (Type D, Type IIIa, Type IIIb,

and Type IV). This can be done manually. However, due to the cartilage roof being pressed caudally, the femoral head cannot immediately be reduced into the acetabulum. The femoral head must at least be placed in front of the entrance to the acetabulum (Fig. 11.1) by directing it medially and caudally. This can be done manually or with a reduction brace, such as the Pavlik harness.

> **Practical tip**
> To direct the femoral head downwards, it is important to position the hip in flexion of about 100–110° and abduction of maximum 60°. This is called the human position. If a Pavlik harness is used for reduction, the straps will prevent leg extension and the forces will direct the femoral head towards the acetabulum for reduction.

Which treatment device is used is irrelevant as long as the basic principle is followed, namely that the treatment device reduces the hip joint

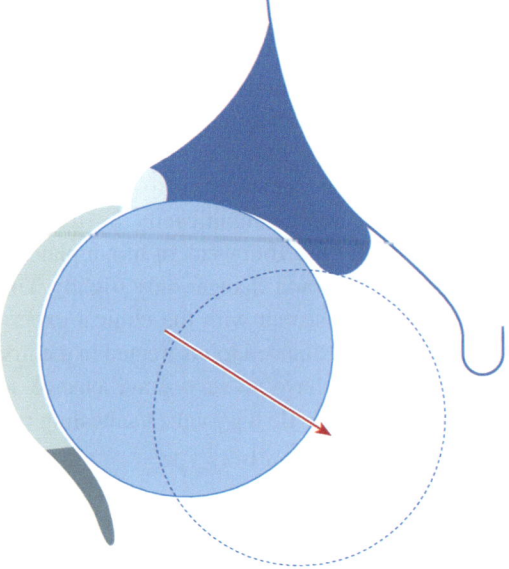

Fig. 11.1 Reduction. The aim of this treatment phase is to position the femoral head at least in front of the constricted, narrow entrance of the acetabulum or, if possible, immediately into the acetabulum

into the centre of the acetabulum. Some reduction devices are better due to their mechanical design, while others are less suitable. However, in principle, it must be a "reduction orthosis" in the broadest sense of the word. Using hip ultrasound as a screening tool, the diagnosis of a hip dislocation is usually nowadays made immediately after birth. As a result, hip maturation disorders are much less severe at the time of diagnosis. As the pathological anatomical changes in the acetabulum are not so severe, immediate manual reduction without a preparatory phase is often possible. With a dynamic sonographic examination using traction, slight abduction, and internal rotation, it can easily be assessed whether primary manual reduction is possible (Fig. 11.2). In some cases, the downwards pressed portion of the hyaline cartilage forming the roof of the acetabulum, can block the reduction of the femoral head into the depth of the acetabulum. The concentric reduction of the femoral head into the acetabulum is a dynamic process in these cases. Through micromovements, the femoral head gently remodels the portion of the roof of the acetabulum that has been pressed caudally, without destroying the

growth area at the chondro-osseous border of the acetabulum.

The longer the hip is decentred, the worse the deformity of the cartilaginous roof, and the more difficult and time-consuming is the restoration to normal morphology for age.

The femoral head must not be pressed forcefully into the acetabulum. Excessive pressure on the femoral head would lead to avascular necrosis caused by the compression of the sinusoids, as well as compression of the cartilaginous acetabular roof that is pushed caudally. For this reason, forced reduction manoeuvres should be avoided, as well as abduction beyond 50–60°, which would also increase axial pressure. The concentric reduction of the femoral head into the depth of the original acetabulum in these cases is a dynamic process, in which the femoral head carefully remodels the caudally displaced hyaline cartilage, through very small micro movements.

Note
From a medical-biomechanical perspective, hip sonography should be performed as early as possible.

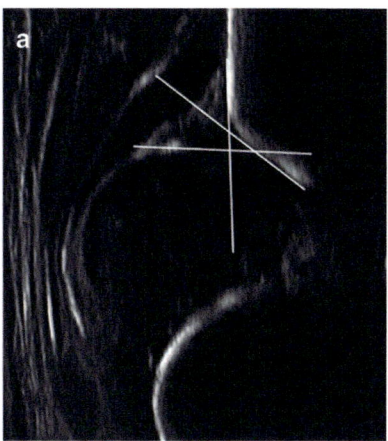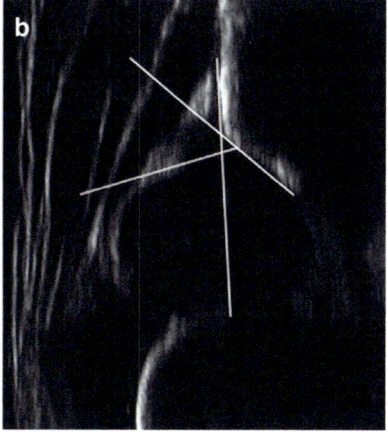

Fig. 11.2 Reduction phase (**a**) Example of a "dynamic" US examination, applying traction to test if reduction is possible. The bony roof is highly deficient, the bony rim is round to flat, and the cartilaginous roof is displaced. The α angle is 48°, and the β angle is 103°. This corresponds to a Type D hip. (**b**) The same hip joint as in (**a**), now under traction to simulate reduction. With the same α angle, the β angle becomes significantly smaller. Also, visually, the hip joint appears centred now. The angle α is 48°, and the angle β is 75°. Hip type under traction measurement: Type IIc

11.4.3 Retention

Once the femoral head is reduced into the acetabulum or at least in front of the entrance of the acetabulum, it is important to maintain this position during the phase of retention. The femoral head tends to re-dislocate into the secondary socket (Fig. 11.3). The joint is unstable.

The principal of treatment must therefore be to hold the femoral head securely in the primary socket. Under no circumstances should the femoral head re-dislocate, as otherwise the resulting compressive and shearing forces prevent the reorganization of the cell columns within the hyaline cartilage roof. Therefore, shearing and compressive forces acting in a cranial direction must be avoided [6], as they would lead to re-dislocation.

Complete Reduction of the Femoral Head
In this phase, the femoral head must be brought into a position that relieves the pressure from the cartilaginous roof. This can be achieved through

complete reduction in a flexion-abduction position (human position). This means fixing the joint in flexion of 100–110°. The stabilization of the femoral head in the socket is achieved through abduction of up to 45–50°, maximum 60°.

With increasing abduction, the femoral head is pressed with greater force in the axial direction into the acetabulum. This makes the femoral head more stable, but it also increases the direct pressure, compressing the sinusoids and potentially causing avascular necrosis.

Immobilization and Time
Stable retention with immobilization of the joint is required. It is understandable that in this delicate retention phase, constant sliding back and forth of the femoral head between the primary and secondary acetabulum, does not allow remodelling nor tightening of the joint capsule [5].

> **Note**
>
> The duration of the retention phase is typically 2–4 weeks, depending on the deformation of the acetabulum and the age of the patient. In older children, it can sometimes be longer.

Hip joints that require secure retention are essentially unstable joints. If the sonographic typing is used, these are joints that were formerly dislocated, such as Type D, Type IIIa, Type IIIb, and Type IV, which have been reduced and are now entering the retention phase, also unstable Type IIc joints.

Treatment in this phase must be performed with a retention orthosis keeping the hip in a flexion-abduction position with full reduction and secure stabilization of the joint. However, it is recommended that a hip spica cast is used for secure retention in worst-case scenarios (parental compliance). This so-called Fettweis cast has been modified so that the lower legs and knee joints are not immobilized (see Fig. 11.4a). As a result, all other joints except the hip joint can move freely. The padding of the cast allows for micro-movements that help nourish the cartilage in the hip joint.

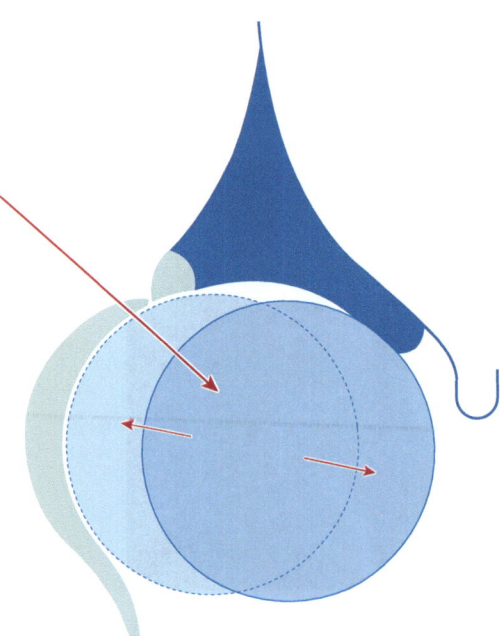

Fig. 11.3 Retention. The hip joint is unstable. Although the femoral head can be reduced, it tends to re-dislocate into the secondary socket. The cartilaginous acetabular roof is still deformed, and the joint capsule is stretched and elongated. The desired position of the femoral head is indicated by the long arrow

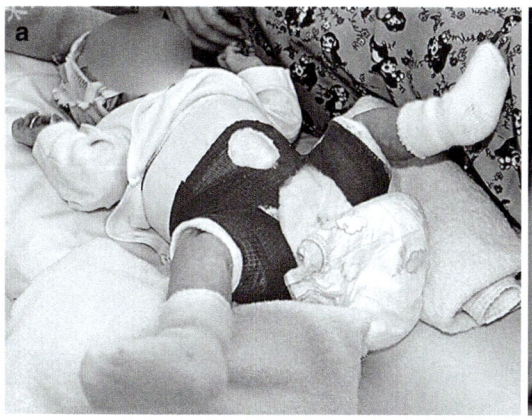
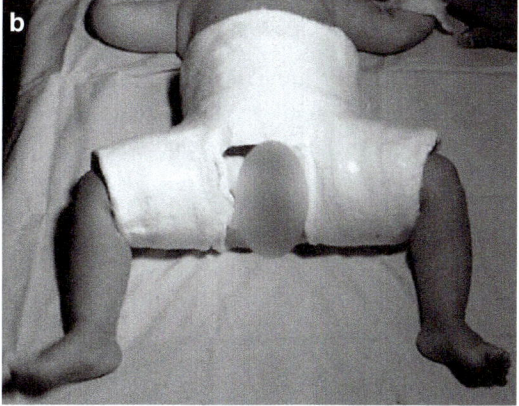

Fig. 11.4 Hip spica cast (**a**) modified so-called Fettweis plaster in the human position (**b**) Lorenz plaster no longer used today with excessive abduction and without flexion (image from 1971)

Unfortunately, for no good reason, casts still have a bad reputation: it must be emphasized that it is not the cast itself that damages the hip joint, but rather the incorrect (Lorenz) position in the cast (see Fig. 11.4b) [5].

> **Learning Point**
>
> An abduction angle of 90° must be avoided with any treatment device!

The plaster cast also has the invaluable advantage that it cannot be altered by parents unlike an adjustable or removable brace. The correct or incorrect position of the femoral head can be seen in Fig. 3.40. The advantage of a correctly applied cast is that it ensures that pathological forces caused by excessive movements, as are possible with retention orthoses, can largely be eliminated.

11.4.4 Maturation Phase

From a patho-anatomical perspective, the femoral head is now deeply seated in the socket, the hyaline cartilaginous roof has regained its original shape and is congruent with the femoral head. The joint capsule is tight, the hip joint is stable, but the cartilaginous roof is not yet sufficiently ossified (see Fig. 11.5).

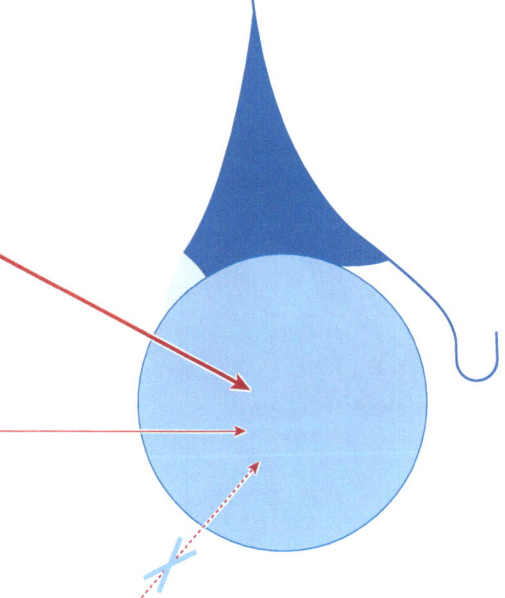

Fig. 11.5 Maturation phase. Cranially directed pressure on the cartilaginous roof must be avoided completely while the reduction of the femoral head is maintained. Micro movements in the joint are permissible while avoiding extension

Pressure and shear forces on the cartilaginous roof in a cranial direction would cause the cartilaginous roof to deform again and cause redislocation. Therefore, further measures to relieve the pressures on the acetabular roof need to be carried out with a prolonged flexion-abduction position [7, 8]. Small movements in the flexion-abduction position are allowed in this phase.

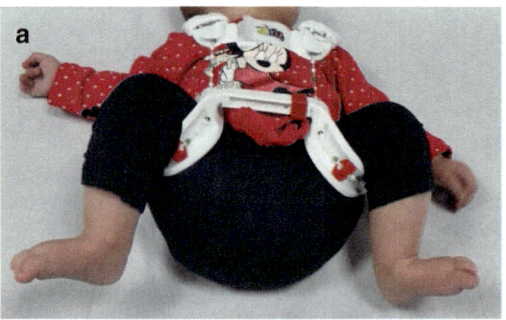

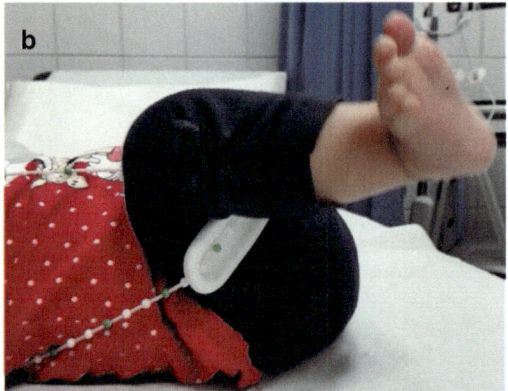

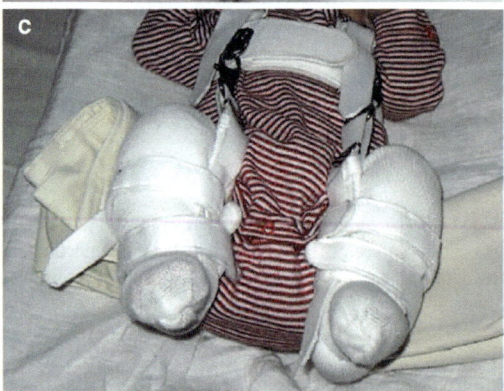

Fig. 11.6 Flexion-abduction position with various braces (**a**) Tübinger brace in flexion-abduction position (**b**) Tübinger brace side view (**c**) Pavlik harness in correct position

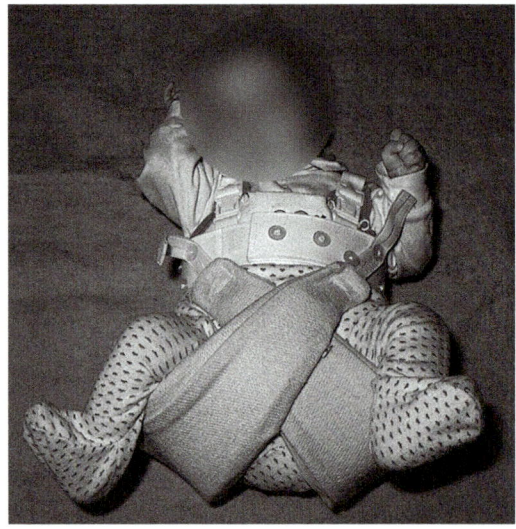

Fig. 11.7 Superior "Spreizhose" as a maturation orthosis. Crossed reins for adjustment in a flexion-abduction position

Maturation is needed for hips that are stable, but not yet fully mature, i.e. not sonographically Type I. These are hip joints of Type IIc stable, Type IIb, and Type IIa -. There are numerous maturation orthoses that allow flexion with moderate abduction and simultaneous kicking movements (Superior, Pavlik, Tübinger, etc.). It is important to maintain the flexion-abduction position (Fig. 11.6 and Fig. 11.7). An overview of the suitable treatment options for each hip type can be found in Table 11.1. An example treatment algorithm is shown in Fig. 11.8.

Table 11.1 Overview of the treatment algorithm with the phases of treatment and the possible treatment methods

Phase	Hip Type	Treatment- method	Alternative Treatment	Remarks
Preparation phase	Type III, Type IV	Overhead extension	–	–
Reduction decentred joints	Type III, Type IV Type D	Manual reduction	Dynamic reduction brace: Pavlik harness	Compliance?
Retention previously decentred, reduced joints, unstable joints	All reduced hips Type IIc - unstable	Hip spica in human position (110°/45°)	Pavlik in correct position for retention	Compliance?
Maturation stable, immature hips	All joints after retention Type IIc – stable Type IIa-, Type IIb	–	Most other flexion/ abduction braces (Superior, Pavlik, Tübinger, Coxa flex)	Braces with more than 60°abduction are outdated

Fig. 11.8 Sonographic documentation of a treatment pathway according to the above illustrated treatment plan

Left Type IV hip diagnosed at newborn screening, application of overhead extension

●

(a) Type III

●

1 week old
After 3 days of extension
Type III
then manual reduction

●

Type IIc stable

●

After reduction and 3 weeks
of retention
Type IIc stable
application of a superior brace

●

(b) Type IIa(-)

●

8 weeks old
after 4 weeks in
superior brace

●

(c) Type Ib

●

15 weeks old
Type Ib

●

End of treatment

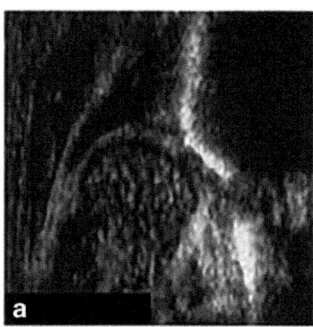

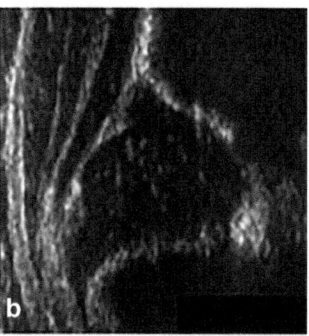

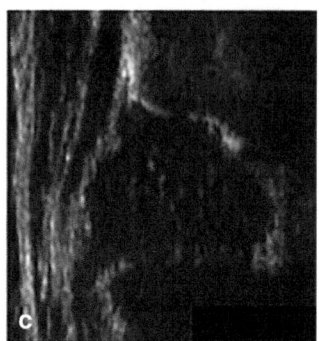

Xray of the left dislocated hip
10 months after treatment

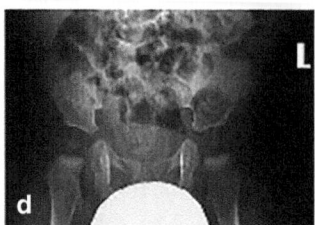

11.5 Deviation from the Treatment Algorithm in Newborns

When newborn hip screening is performed, Type D and Type III joints are often still in the standard plane. The proportion of these joints in newborn screening accounts for up to 77% of all hip joints requiring treatment [9]. In addition, when a hip dislocation is diagnosed in early infancy, the entire exponential growth phase within the hip maturation curve [1] can be made use of for the time of treatment. Due to the combination of a more favourable initial situation and a high potential for remodelling, the treatment recommendations for newborns increasingly deviate from those for older infants.

In cases of early diagnosis, dislocated hip joints that are still in the standard plane can often be successfully reduced and retained using the easily manageable hip flexion orthoses approved for post-maturation treatment [10]. A prerequisite for this is that the parents have a good understanding of the necessary treatment steps to ensure the high compliance that is required. Hip flexion orthoses should only be removed temporarily for nappy changes and hygiene measures for the entire duration of treatment. The minimum daily time in the brace should be 23 h.

Furthermore, this type of treatment requires an initial sonographic follow-up examination after 1 week, or at the latest after 14 days. If there is no improvement or even deterioration, a change of treatment plan to closed reduction and retention of the joint using a hip spica cast should be made at this point, in consideration of the remodelling potential within the early part of the hip maturation curve (Table 11.2). A deterioration of findings is indicated with the inability to visualize the femoral head in the standard plane and the inability to reduce the hip joint. An example of sonographic monitoring with reduction is shown in Fig. 11.9.

Various working groups [11–15] were able to demonstrate that this treatment option can also be effective for Type IV joints and older infants. Accordingly, the S2k guideline "Hip Dysplasia", recommends that in babies under 6 weeks of age, when the initial diagnosis is of hip subluxation, with the standard plane still visible and no clinical signs of instability, parents should be offered a trial of treatment with a hip flexion orthosis as an alternative to applying a spica cast or a Pavlik harness (hip Type D, if applicable, hip Type III). In babies under 6 weeks of age with an initial diagnosis of hip subluxation without being able to visualize the hip joint in the standard plane (hip Type IV, if applicable,

Table 11.2 Treatment recommendations at the time of initial diagnosis of hip dysplasia in newborns

Treatment phase	Hip Type	Treatment	Alternative treatment
Reduction	Type IV Type III, no longer in the standard plane	Manual closed reduction	Pavlik Harness, Trial of Tübinger Brace for max 14 days
	Type III, still in the standard plane Type D	Tübinger Brace, if not reduced within 14 days proceed to manual closed reduction	Pavlik Harness
Retention	Manually reduced Type IV Manually reduced Type III	Hip spica in human position	Pavlik Harness
	Hips successfully reduced with Tübinger Brace, Type III, Type D, Type IIc unstable	Tübinger Brace	Hip spica Pavlik Harness
Maturation	All joints after retention Type IIc stable, Type IIb, Type IIa-	Abduction brace (E.g. continue with Tübinger Brace)	Pavlik Harness

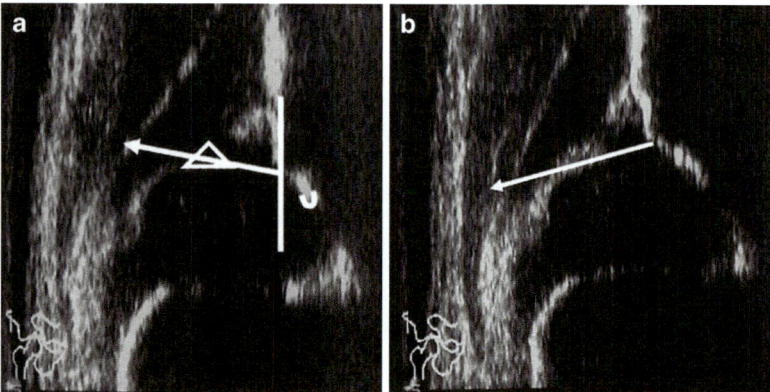

Fig. 11.9 Example of reduction (**a**) Initial diagnosis of a dislocated hip joint at the age of 4 weeks with cranially displaced cartilaginous roof (arrow) but still visible in the standard plane with the lower limb (arc), plane (line), and labrum (triangle) all visible (**b**) Reduction of the previously dislocated hip joint within 9 days in the Tübinger orthosis with the cartilaginous roof line now pointing downwards (arrow)

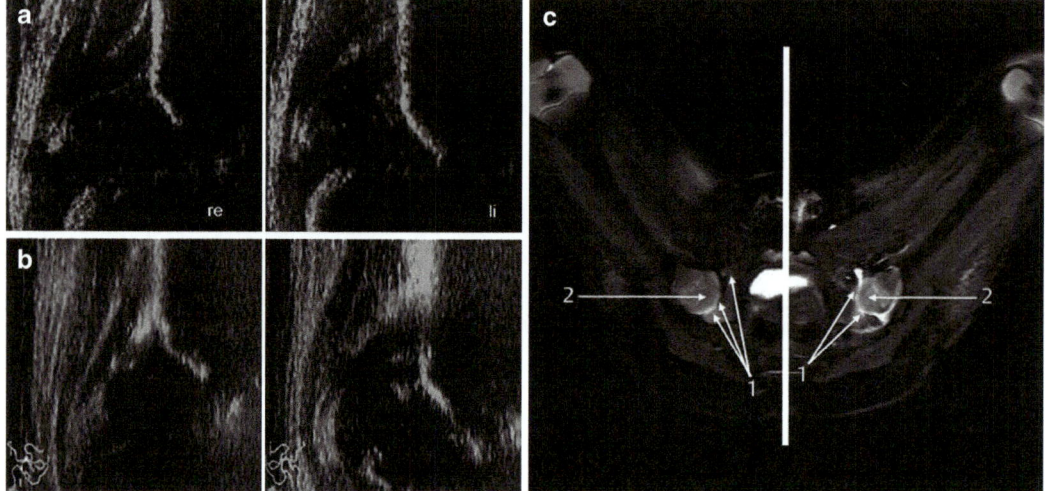

Fig. 11.10 Reduction and retention using the Tübinger splint for bilateral hip dislocation (li = left re = right, (**a**) Hip ultrasound findings at 2 days of age. Right Type III maintained in the standard plane), (left Type IV. (**b**) Hip ultrasound findings after 2 weeks of treatment with the Tübinger splint. Right Type IIa with bony rim defect, left persistent Type IV. (**c**) MRI control after closed reduction under anaesthesia and application of hip spica cast. Hips reduced on both sides, the acetabulum on the left is still much too small for the femoral head compared to the right. 1 = acetabulum. (2 = femoral head)

hip Type III) as well as in cases where the joint is still visible in the standard plane, but with clinically detectable instability, the treating physician can offer a treatment trial with a hip flexion orthosis, with an obligation to obtain specific consent and provide appropriate information. Fig. 11.10 shows the classic course of bilateral hip dislocation diagnosed in the first week of life during attempted reduction and retention using a Tübinger brace.

11.6   Treatment Failures

The fact that there can ultimately be poor treatment outcomes despite all efforts is mainly based, as error analyses have shown, on the following three problem areas.

11.6.1   Late Diagnosis with Subsequent Delayed Start of Treatment

The hip joint matures very well in the first 4—6 weeks. The growth potential clearly plateaus towards the end of the third month of life. The earlier the diagnosis is made, the earlier the treatment can begin, and the maturation potential can be utilized. Also for organizational reasons treatment is started preferably as early as possible after birth the window for diagnosis and commencement of treatment closes at the latest in the fifth week of life [6].

> **Remember**
> Motto of diagnosis and treatment in DDH:
>
> - "Don't waste time."
> - "To screen or not to screen is not the question—it's politics!"

11.6.2   Inappropriate Choice of Treatment for the Stage

One major problem occurs if a treatment modality is chosen that simply cannot provide the function needed for the respective patho-anatomical situation, i.e. the respective sonographic type. For example, a "Spreizhose" is a typical treatment modality for the stage of maturation. It cannot perform a reduction nor can it maintain a reduction due to its biomechanical design.

The concept of treatment stages with reduction, retention, further maturation, and the recommended methods of treatment are usually safe

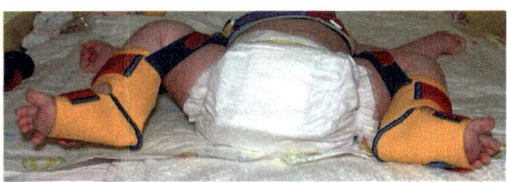

Fig. 11.11   Lorenz position with 90° hip flexion and 90° abduction in the Pavlik harness. However, it is essential to avoid 90° abduction to prevent avascular necrosis of the femoral head

even in the worst-case scenario. Exceptions can only be made in newborns.

11.6.3   Lack of Parental Compliance

Undoubtedly, a hip joint in need of treatment represents a significant psychological burden for the parents of the child.

The treatment device that seems most comfortable to the parents is often not the most effective one for the hip joint. The retention phase is biomechanically the most sensitive: Any treatment device that is questionable in maintaining retention, i.e. can be removed and adjusted by the parents, or manipulated in any other way, poses a great risk. In cases when the compliance of the parents is doubtful ("doctor-shopping", seeking information on the internet), cast immobilization in a flexion-abduction position is recommended. If removable treatment devices are used, such as the Pavlik harness, it must be ensured that it is not only adjusted to the size of the child, but also adapted to the treatment phase. The treating healthcare professional must also ensure that the family members understand not to remove the orthosis out of misguided pity. Potentially they might either not reapply it at all or apply it in a wrong position Fig. 11.11.

11.7   Follow-up Intervals

According to the growth potential of the hip joint, for hip joints requiring treatment that are younger than 3 months, the sonographic follow-up interval should be set at 4–6 weeks. In infants, older than 3 months, hip maturation slows down significantly, so a follow-up interval of 8–10 weeks is recommended.

11.8 Summary

Conclusion

- Rules:
  - Treat immediately according to the stage, do not "try out" different devices.
  - Each sonographic type can be assigned to one of the three treatment phases.
  - In each treatment phase, a specific orthosis is biomechanically effective.
  - The most delicate treatment phase is the retention phase: a stable and secure reduction of the hip joint is necessary. All devices that can be adjusted or removed by parents (compliance) pose a risk.
- Exceptions: Possible in newborns.

References

1. Tschauner C, Klapsch W, Baumgartner A et al. "Reifungskurve" des sonographischen Alpha-Winkels nach Graf un- behandelter Hüftgelenke im ersten Lebensjahr. Z Orthop 1994; 132: 502–504.
2. Graf R. Sonographie der Säuglingshüfte. Ein Kompendium. 4th ed. Stuttgart: Enke; 1993.
3. Merk H, Mahlfeld K, Wissel H, et al. The congenital dislocation of the hip joint in ultrasound examination—frequency, diagnosis and treatment. Klin Padiatr. 1992;211:18–21.
4. Graf R, Hammer N, Matthiesen D. An integrated concept explaining for risk factors related to the onset of develop- mental dysplasia of the hip joint. Ann Orthop Musculo- skelet Disord. 2021;4(1):1029.
5. Tönnis D. Die angeborene Hüftdysplasie und Hüftluxation im Kindes- und Erwachsenenalter. Berlin: Springer; 1984.
6. Matthiessen HD. Dysplasie- und Therapiefaktor bei der Hüftreifungsstörung. Z Orthop. 1997;135:12–3.
7. Fettweis E. Sitz-Hock-Stellungsgips bei Hüftgelenksdysplasien. Arch Orthop Trauma Surg. 1968;63:38–51.
8. Fettweis E. Das kindliche Hüftluxationsleiden. Die Behand- lung in Sitz-Hock-Stellung (mit umfangreicher Bibliographie). Landsberg/Lech: ecomed; 1992.
9. Seidl T, Lohmaier J, Trouillier HH. Früherkennung der Hüftdysplasie. Monatsschr Kinderheilkd. 2011;159:758–61.
10. Seidl T, Lohmaier J, Hölker T, et al. Die Tübinger Hüftbeugeschiene als Repositionsorthese? Orthopade. 2012;41:195–9.
11. Atalar H, Gunay C, Komurcu M. Functional treatment of developmental hip dysplasia with the Tübingen hip flexion splint. Hip Int. 2014;24:295–301.
12. Kubo H, Pilge H, Weimann-Stahlschmidt K, et al. Use of the Tübingen splint for the initial management of severly dysplastic and unstable hips in newborns with DDH: an alternative to Fettweis plaster and Pavlik harness. Arch Orthop Trauma Surg. 2018;138:149–53.
13. Munkhuu B, Essig S, Renchinnyam E, et al. Incidence and treatment of developmental hip dysplasia in Mongolia: a prospective cohort study. PLoS One. 2013;8(e79):427.
14. Pavone V, Testa G, Riccioli M, et al. Treatment of develop- mental dysplasia of hip with Tubingen hip flexion splint. J Pediatr Orthop. 2015;35:485–9.
15. Ulziibat M, Munkhuu B, Schmid R, et al. Implementation of a nationwide universal ultrasound screening programme for developmental dysplasia of the neonatal hip in mongo- lia. J Child Orthop. 2020;14:273–80.

Course Programme and Syllabus

12

The course syllabus is intended to help trainers in hip sonography. It should enable a systematic training structure with completion of the educational content. In addition, it should provide tips and tricks on common mistakes and how to avoid them.

12.1 Fundamentals of Hip Sonography

Basics of hip sonography are shown in Table 12.1.

Table 12.1 Fundamentals of hip sonography

Syllabus	Comments, Tips and Tricks
Order of checklists	Checklist I always before checklist II
Anatomical identification (Checklist I)	Important: Always start with the anatomical identification, then continue with usability check – never the other way around! Otherwise, a decentred hip could be overlooked as the lower limb is missing in decentred joints because the femoral head is not always in the standard plane
Usability check (Checklist II) including check for tilting mistakes	• Lower limb • Plane • Labrum
Scanning technique	A good scanning technique shortens the examination time, which indirectly improves the quality of the sonogram (baby not moving) making the Identification and usability checks possible

12.2   Anatomical Identification

Anatomical landmarks are summarized in Table 12.2.

> **Practical tip**
>
> **Checklist I**
>   All structures of Checklist I must be visualized on the sonogram. If even one structure is missing, the sonogram should not be accepted for diagnosis.

Table 12.2 Anatomical identification. Note: For the anatomical identification, always start with the chondro-osseous border

Anatomical landmarks	Comments, tips and tricks
Chondro-osseous border	• mention the 3 typical shapes (curved, with sound palisades, and angular)
Femoral head	• head is not round, explain sinusoids and their significance (zona anularis, zona centralis)
	• ossific nucleus: not in the centre, not round, visible 4-8 weeks earlier in ultrasound than in X-ray, half-moon phenomenon
	• explain problems with a large ossific nucleus (limits the method, no size determination possible)
Synovial fold	• easily confused with the labrum
	• representation as an echogenic spot or 2 parallel echoes
Joint capsule	• echo corresponds to the capsule and not the surface of the femoral head
Labrum	• 4 definitions of the labrum to locate it in every case, even if it is poorly visible
	• do not confuse with the lig. ischiofemorale
Standard sequence	• standard sequence for the safe identification of the cartilage roof (often forgotten or incorrectly identified)
	• bone: follow the os ilium from "top" to "bottom" to the lower edge of the os ilium, then determine the turning point (see below)
Turning point	• definition: concavity - convexity = turning point
	• always search for the turning point from "bottom" to "top" (can be identified precisely lateral to the acoustic shadow)
	• localization of the "corner" of the curve: example sinus curve with turning point of the two opposite curves ("concavity to convexity")

Lig. = Ligamentum

12.3   Usability Check

The usability check is described in Table 12.3.

Practical tip
Checklist II
  Usability check:

- Three points define a plane in 3D space.
- The order corresponds to the importance of structures visualised: lower limb–plane–labrum. Credo: always perform anatomical identification first, then usability check and a check for tilting errors, never the other way around.
- If anatomical identification is performed first, it can be determined whether it is a centred joint or not. This puts the usability check in context and explains the absence of the lower limb of the ilium in decentred hips.
- If the usability check is done first, a decentred hip may be overlooked if the lower limb of the ilium is missing and the sonogram is incorrectly dismissed.

Conclusion
Anatomical identification and usability check

- Landmarks:
  - chondro-osseous border.
  - femoral head.
  - synovial fold.
  - joint capsule.
  - labrum–cartilage–bone.
  - concavity–convexity with turning point.
  - lower limb.
  - plane.
  - labrum.
- Do not use a sonogram if only one of these points cannot be identified.
- Exception: decentred hips.

Table 12.3 Usability check

Anatomical landmarks	Course work
Lower limb of os ilium	The lower limb is the sonographic centre of the acetabulum. It is the axis of rotation for the plane. Thus, the lower limb is the most important reference point of the standard plane and takes priority over the plane through the acetabular roof and the labrum. "If the lower limb is not visible, hip sonography is dead". Exception: In dislocated joints, the lower limb may be absent because the femoral head has dislocated dorsocranially and left the standard plane.
Plane	(anterior, middle, posterior plane) The echo silhouette of the plane should be drawn. The explanation why the dorsal bony rim of the acetabulum is better developed than the middle and anterior parts is based on evolutionary development. Only the middle plane may be used. Exception: In dislocated joints. In the case of dorsocranial dislocation, the dorsal plane is also possible on the sonogram: • Assessment and classification are possible in this case, • Measurement is not possible, because it is not in the standard plane and measurements can only be obtained in the standard plane.
Labrum	By visualizing the labrum as a third point, oblique cross sections (tilts) are avoided. If the labrum is scanned too obliquely, the reflective conditions are so poor that it is not visible.

12.4   Hip Types

Differentiation between hip types, see Table 12.4.

Table 12.4 Description of hip types from Type I to Type IV. They can be demonstrated in sonograms but drawings are more schematic and easy to understand for the novice

Type	Description
I	• Mature joint, expected by the end of 12th week • The term "Mature" is better than "healthy" (a Type-IIa+ hip is also healthy) • The difference between Type Ia and Type Ib should only be explained in the context of α and β angles (p.125)
II	• Delayed ossification: The femoral head is overall covered, the proportion of coverage has shifted in favour of the cartilaginous cover
III and IV	• Type III: decentred joints; hyaline cartilage mostly pushed upward, only a small portion pressed downward • Type IV: entire acetabular hyaline cartilage pushed downward, towards the true socket (original acetabulum); no acetabular hyaline cartilage visible above the femoral head • Sonographic differentiation of Type III and Type IV hips: differentiation between Type III and Type IV in the sonogram is based on the direction of the perichondrium, not on the position of the labrum • Subluxation is a clinical term, "a little dislocated", it is incorrect to refer to Type III as subluxation.

12.5 Reporting

The information that has to be in the US report is summarized in Table 12.5.

Table 12.5 Standard reporting

Standards	Course content
Standardised sonogram	• Age
	• Description
	• α/β angle and final type (measuring technique see Table 12.7)
	• Treatment consequences
Standardised report	• Patient identification, side
	• 2 sonograms in the standard plane at different times, one with measurement lines, one without measurement lines
	• Picture size of at least 1.7:1 for paper printouts

12.6 Description

The description allows preliminary Typing (estimate) and requires correct anatomical identification to estimate the proportions of the coverage (Table 12.6). The final verification is done through measurements. In the case of a discrepancy between the description and the measurements, both the description, is the anatomical identification correct? and the measurement lines need to be checked. The findings must correspond.

Table 12.6 Description

Conceptual terms	Course content
Reporting and terminology for the bony roof, the bony rim, and the cartilaginous coverage.	By differentiating bony coverage with the help of the turning point into "more than half" or "less than half" and assessing the level of the labrum in relation to the turning point, Types I, II, and III can be roughly differentiated. However, all measurement techniques that are based on bony coverage are only estimates: To estimate "half," one needs the centre of the femoral head, but it cannot be determined reproducibly as the femoral head is not round. Therefore, all measurement techniques that use the centre of the femoral head are only estimates.
Ongoing maturation/Remodelling	Ongoing maturation can be explained as development of an angular acetabular rim instead of a rounded one in type II joints. It should also be explained how a potential discrepancy between a sonogram and an Xray can occur (time difference).

12.7   Measurement Technique

Table 12.7 shows how the measurement lines are to be drawn.

Learning point

- Only sonograms in the standard plane may be measured, without exception.
- All three lines only intersect at one point in a classic Type-I hip with an angular bony rim. However, this is quite rare, so always be cautious when all three measurement lines intersect at one point.

Table 12.7 Drawing of the measurement lines

Measurement lines	Course content
Bony roof line	• The bony roof line is drawn from the lower limb (as a pivot point), tangential to, just touching, the bony roof. • Tangential to the bony roof does not mean that the line goes through the turning point • At the lower limb, the echoes that can lead to misinterpretation should be explained: – Sinusoids in the triradiate cartilage, – Fat tissue.
Baseline	• The baseline is drawn from the topmost point of the attachment of the proximal perichondrium to the os ilium (Z-point), downwards tangential to, just touching, the os ilium. • Most of the proximal perichondrium consists of the rectus tendon, so the attachment area (Z-point) is actually the origin of the rectus tendon.
Cartilage roof line	• Is drawn from the turning point (concavity – convexity) through the centre of the labrum. • Centre of the labrum means the main echo. • The turning point is rarely the intersection of the baseline and bony roof line. This only occurs where the bony rim is sharply angular

12.8   Sonometer

The cartilage and bony roof angles are explained
Table 12.8.

> **Learning point**
>
> The α-angle determines the type, while the
> β-angle allows for differentiation between
> sub-types. Exception: if α falls within the
> Type IIc range, the β-angle determines
> whether it is a Type IIc or a Type D.

Table 12.8   Cartilage and bony roof angles

Terminology	Course content
Explanation of the α-angle values:	• ≥ 60° = Type I (60° is the lowest acceptable value for Type-I hip joints.) • < 43° = decentred joints (Whether it is Type III or Type IV is distinguished morphologically, not by measurement.) • 43–59° = Type-II Range

• Type-II	• Stepwise approach:
	  – Delayed ossification = Type II
	  – Severely delayed ossification; the hip joint will not recover spontaneously and is at risk of decentring if left untreated = Type IIc (43–49°); immediate treatment required
	  – 50–59° = Type IIa or Type IIb
	• Explain correlation with age: physiologically immature hip (Type IIa +) and true ossification deficit (Type IIa–/Type IIb)

• Type IIa+ and Type IIa–	• Explanation based on the timeline from birth to the end of week 12 (To be on the safe side development is considered as linear rather than according to the maturation curve,.)
Explanation of the β-angle values:	• The cartilage roof can have different shapes, with an identical bony roof in Type-I joints

• Type Ia and Type Ib	• Type I hips with a long cartilage roof and β-angle ≤55° = Type Ia
	• Short cartilage roof with β-angle > 55° = Type Ib
	• Type Ia and Type Ib: Variations of a healthy hip joint (like blonde hair/black hair)
	• Type Ib more common and not worse than Type Ia
	• Possible consequences (hypothesis):
	  – Long cartilage roof - possible later impingement
	  – Short cartilage roof - possible early onset of pathological acetabular loading with labral degeneration and tears

• Type IIc and D	• Explanation based on a β-value of 77°

12.9 Instability and Elastic Whipping

The definitions of the terms are noted in Table 12.9.

Learning point

- The term instability summarizes all pathological movements in the hip joint..
- Elastic whipping refers to harmless physiological movements that do not require treatment.

Table 12.9 Definition of the terms "instability" and "elastic whipping"

Terminologies	Course content
Instability	
Definition	The term "Instability" encompasses all pathological movements in the hip joint.
Type IIc – stable and Type IIc – unstable	• It must be explained how type D is determined • The classification Type IId is incorrect, because all Type II joints are centred, but Type D represents the first stage of a decentred hip. • All decentred joints – Type D and worse – are sonographically unstable. • Explanation of the developmental dislocation process: As soon as the α angle is in the Type IIc range, the shear forces at the chondro-osseous border of the acetabular growth plate increase to such an extent, that endochondral ossification ceases (growth arrest), and a progressive flattening of the acetabular roof occurs, leading to dislocation of the femoral head, which can no longer be kept within the acetabulum.
Elastic whipping	
Definition	• Summary of all physiological movements in the hip joint: Elastic whipping includes the up and down movement of the labrum or hyaline acetabular cartilage, during rotational movements, due to the physiological incongruence of the femoral head and the acetabulum or a loose joint capsule.
Transition from (physiological) elastic whipping to (pathological) instability	• ≥ 50°: Elastic whipping • < 50°: The α angle is in the Type IIc range; this is considered instability.

12.10 Tilting Errors

Tilting errors (Table 12.10) can lead to misdiagnoses. Causes:

- Defraction and refraction with image distortion due to the oblique sound beam.
- Loss of important landmarks.

Practical tip

Tilting errors can only be minimized through appropriate examination techniques or technical equipment (cradle, probe guide).

Table 12.10 Tilting mistakes

Tilting errors	Course content
Ventro-dorsal tilt	
Dorso-ventral tilt	Draw the typical sonographic changes or show examples on sonograms
Cranio-caudal tilt	
Caudo-cranial tilt	

12.11 Scanning Technique

The technical requirements are presented in Table 12.11.

Practical tip

- Always start with the lower limb, never try to visualize the plane first.
- Evaluate the frozen image (stop!) to assess the plane.
- Say the keyword rotate under visual control, then turn the transducer in the correct direction and show the lower limb again.
- Make sure that the examiner switches between looking at the monitor and looking at the ultrasound probe.

Table 12.11   Scanning technique (www.graf-hipsonography.com).

Examination steps	Explanations and course content
Technical requirements:	
• Examination table and cradle	• Scanning technique has nothing to do with experience or skill. The step-by-step technique has to be practiced on a phantom (driving school).
• Probe guide	• The use of a probe guide is highly recommended to avoid tilting errors.
• Linear transducer with ≥ 5 MHz	
• Documentation template	
Preparation:	• e.g.: "Hello, Mrs. M., please place your right hand on the baby's shoulder..."
• Instructing the parent with clear language	• Ensure a calm atmosphere.
	• Instruct the parent to remove their baby's nappy before entering the examination room.
• Positioning of the child and the transducer	• In the examination room, an additional tray or examination table should be provided for further clinical examination.
	• Begin with the right hip joint. After slightly rotating the leg inward, proceed as follows: – Apply gel directly to the skin, not on the transducer, – Pay attention to finger position, do not flex, – Finger, – Transducer (practice the position!), – Hand.
Examination procedure:	
• forward – backward – forward – backward – smaller – smaller – smaller – stop	• One should focus only on the lower limb of the os ilium and not try to visualize the plane first.
	• With the image frozen, take time to consider in which direction the transducer must be rotated.
• "Search for the lower limb"	
• Rotate further	• When rotating the plane one should look at the transducer, not at the monitor, to ensure rotation in the correct direction.
• forward – backward – forward – backward – smaller – smaller – smaller – stop	• Due to the correction of the plane, the lower limb is lost; therefore, the lower limb must be searched for again.
	• If necessary, the process should be repeated.
• Search for the lower limb	• All other important parts of the image will present themselves automatically with this technique.

Practical Exercises

13

This chapter, through visual material, is intended to support familiarization with hip ultrasound and a systematic approach to interpretation. It is meant to benefit both beginners and those who wish to refresh their knowledge of the sonographic diagnosis of infant hips.

13.1 Part 1: Questions

13.1.1 Identification of Anatomical Structures

See Figs. 13.1, 13.2, 13.3, 13.4, 13.5.

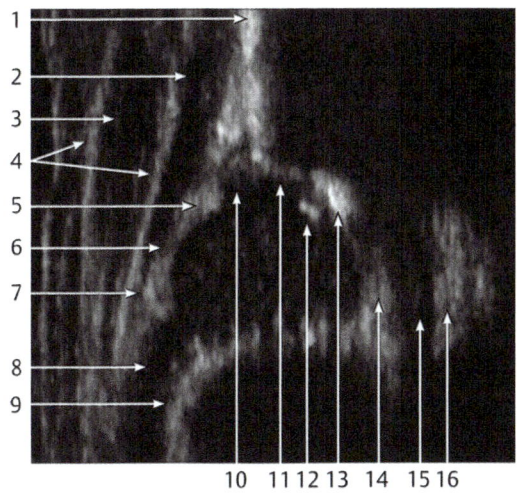

Fig. 13.1 Task 1. Identify the anatomical structures marked on this sonogram

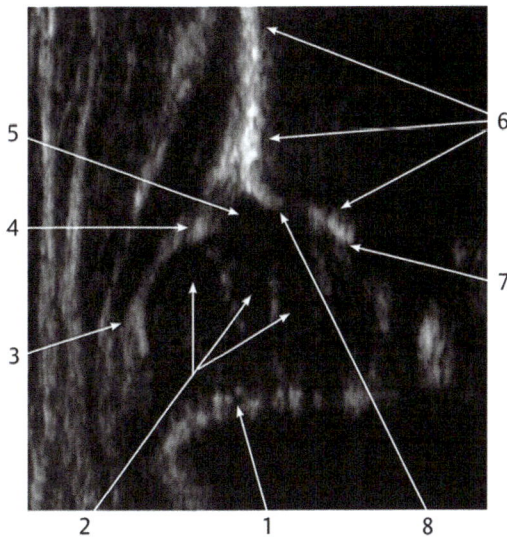

Fig. 13.2 Task 2. Identify the anatomical structures marked on this sonogram

13.1.2 Usability Check (Lower Limb, Plane, Labrum)

See Figs. 13.6, 13.7, 13.8, 13.9, 13.10, 13.11, 13.12, 13.13, 13.14

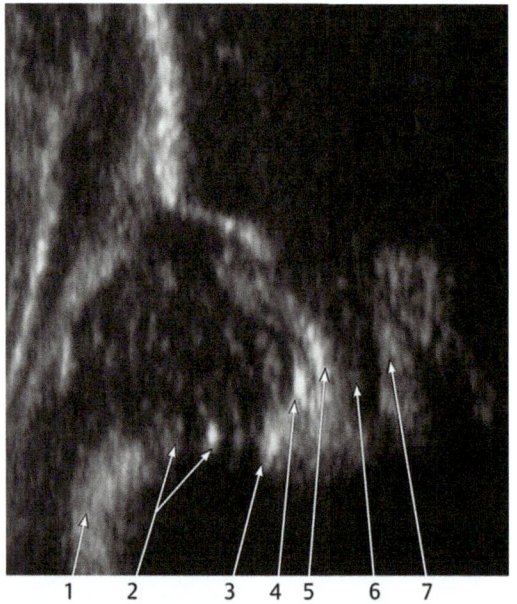

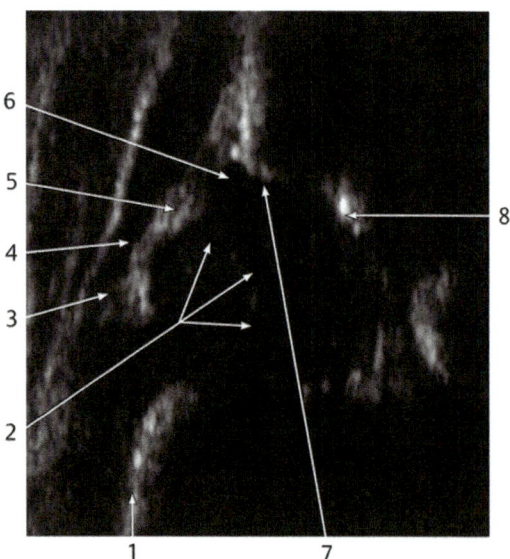

Fig. 13.5 Task 5. Identify the anatomical structures marked on this sonogram

Fig. 13.3 Task 3. Identify the anatomical structures marked on this sonogram

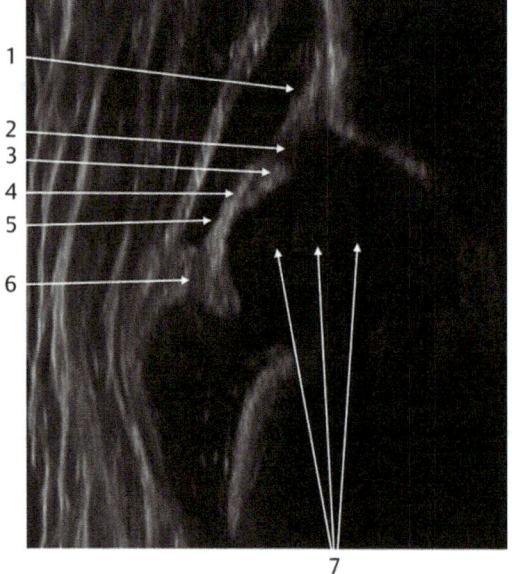

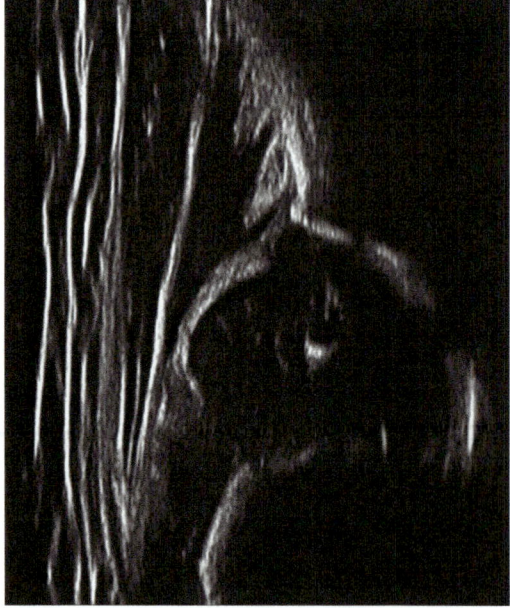

Fig. 13.4 Task 4. Identify the anatomical structures marked on this sonogram

Fig. 13.6 Exercise 6. Was this sonogram taken in the standard plane? If not, which plane could it be?

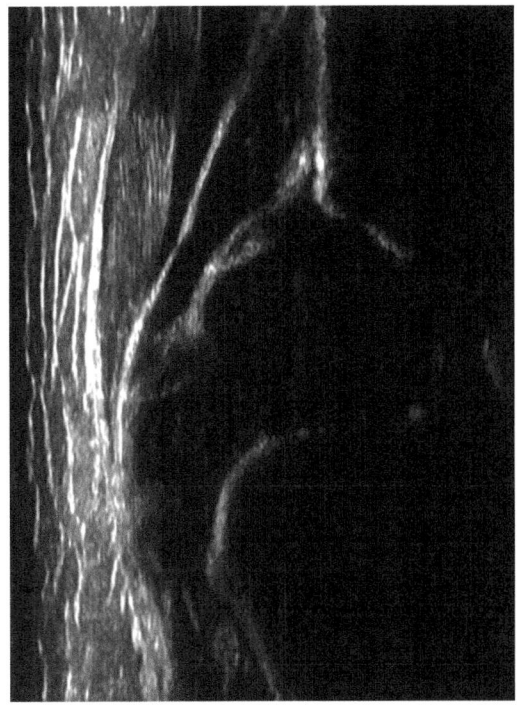

Fig. 13.7 Exercise 7. Is this sonogram usable? If not, why?

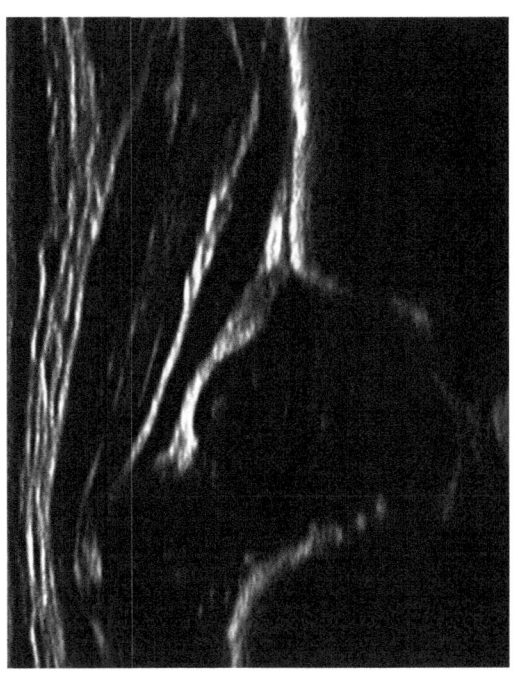

Fig. 13.9 Exercise 9. Is this sonogram usable? If not, why? If yes, why?

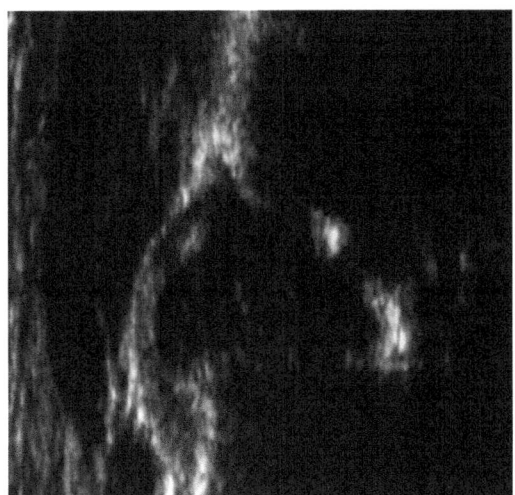

Fig. 13.8 Exercise 8. Is this sonogram usable? If not, why?

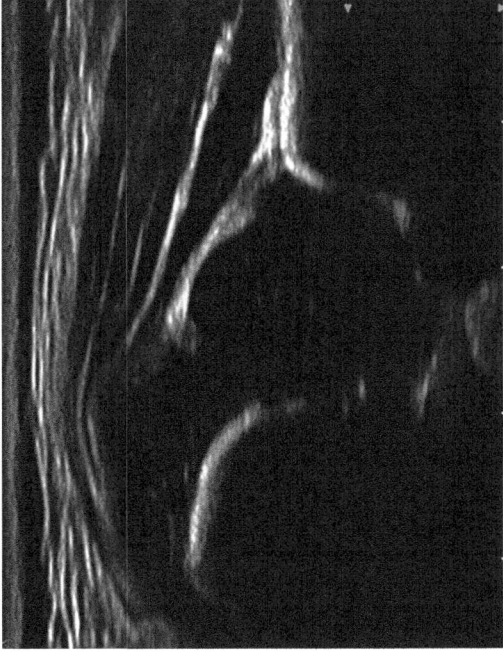

Fig. 13.10 Task 10. The right hip of an 11-week-old child is shown. Task: description and classification

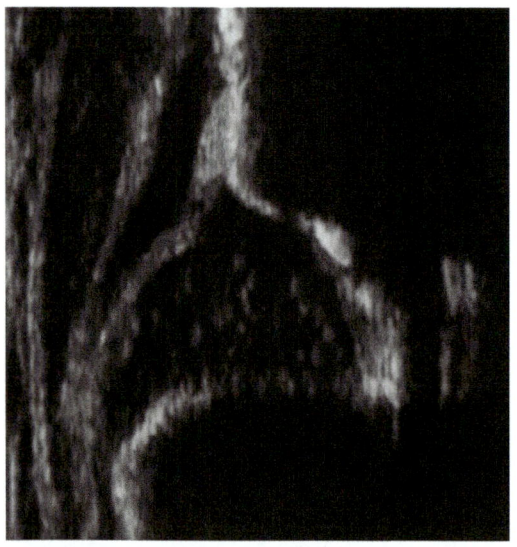

Fig. 13.11 Exercise 11. The left hip of a 3-week-old child is shown. Task: description, angle measurement, and classification

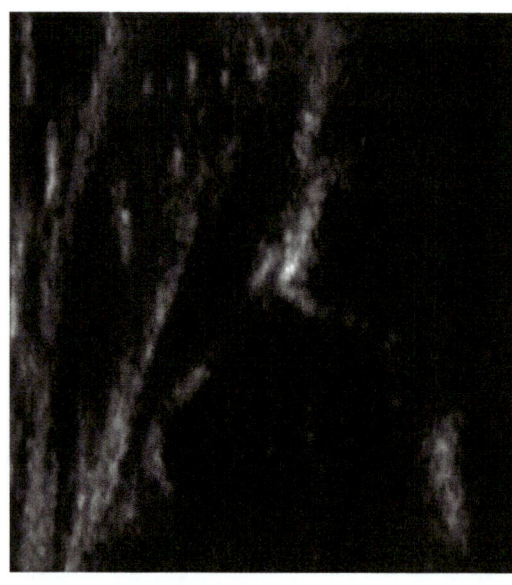

Fig. 13.13 Exercise 13. The left hip of a 3-month-old child is shown. Task: description, angle measurement, and classification

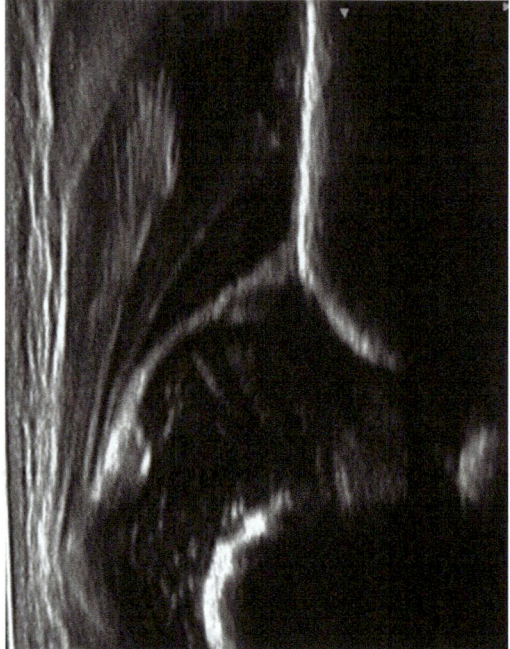

Fig. 13.12 Exercise 12. The right hip of a 2-week-old child is shown. Task: description, angle measurement, and classification

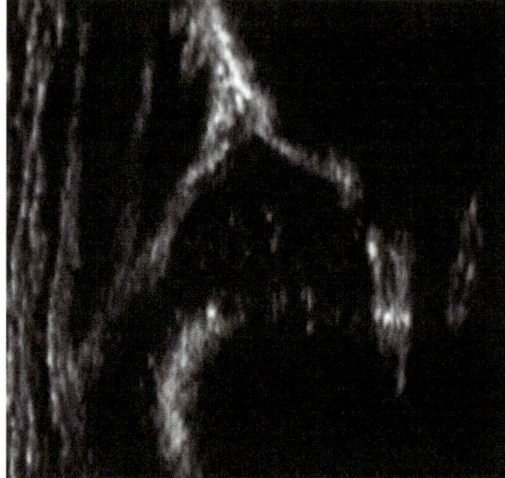

Fig. 13.14 Task 14. The right hip of a 3-week-old child is shown. Does this hip meet the required minimum level of maturity?

13.2   Part 2: Answers

13.2.1 Identification of Anatomical Structures

Exercise 1
1. = os ilium
2. = gluteus minimus muscle
3. = gluteus medius muscle
4. = intermuscular septum
5. = acetabular labrum
6. = joint capsule
7. = synovial fold
8. = cartilaginous greater trochanter
9. = chondro-osseous border
10. = cartilaginous acetabular roof
11. = turning point
12. = ligamentum teres
13. = lower limb of os ilium
14. = perichondrium
15. = triradiate cartilage
16. = perichondrium

Exercise 2
1. = chondro-osseous border
2. =hyaline cartilage of the femoral head
3. = transverse ligament
4. = labrum, more lateral to it is the ischiofemoral ligament
5. = hyaline cartilage of the acetabular roof
6. = bony contour (os ilium and bony roof)
7. = lower limb
8. = turning point

Exercise 3
1. = chondro-osseous border
2. = echo palisades of the chondro-osseous border
3. = transverse ligament
4. = lig. Teres
5. = pulvinar
6. = triradiate cartilage
7. = perichondrium on inner side.

Exercise 4
1. = rectus tendon
2. = perichondrial gap
3. = labrum
4. = ischiofemoral ligament
5. = joint capsule
6. = synovial fold
7. = sinusoids.

Exercise 5
1. = chondro-osseous border
2. = femoral head
3. = synovial fold
4. = joint capsule
5. = labrum
6. = cartilaginous acetabular roof
7. = turning point
8. = lower limb.

13.2.2 Usability Check (Lower Limb, Plane, Labrum)

Exercise 6
This sonogram was not taken in the standard plane. The plane is too ventral.

Exercise 7
This sonogram meets the quality criteria:

• lower limb clearly identifiable,
• correct plane,
• labrum clearly visible.

Exercise 8
During the sonographic examination, the ultrasound probe was tilted in a ventrodorsal direction. This can be recognized in the sonogram by the widening of the silhouette of the os ilium.

Exercise 9
The image is correct:

- The lower limb is clearly identifiableThe silhouette of the ilium is straight
- The labrum is clearly visible.

Exercise 10
The bony roof is good, the bony rim area is angular, and the cartilaginous acetabular roof is covering. This corresponds to a Type I.

Exercise 11
The bony roof is adequate, the bony rim is round, and the cartilaginous roof is covering. The α angle is 55°, and the β angle is 75°. This indicates a Type IIa + .

Exercise 12
The bony roof is poor, the bony rim is flat, and the cartilaginous roof is displaced cranially without structural changes. The hip joint is classified as Type IIIa. It is not possible to measure the angles in this image as the lower limb is not clearly visible.

Exercise 13
This image is not usable:

- The lower limb is missing
- The plane is too posterior
- The labrum is not visible.

Exercise 14
The plane is too far anterior, the sonogram is unusable, and the question regarding the minimum required maturity cannot be answered.

GPSR Compliance

The European Union's (EU) General Product Safety Regulation (GPSR) is a set of rules that requires consumer products to be safe and our obligations to ensure this.

If you have any concerns about our products, you can contact us on ProductSafety@springernature.com

In case Publisher is established outside the EU, the EU authorized representative is:

Springer Nature Customer Service Center GmbH
Europaplatz 3
69115 Heidelberg, Germany

Batch number: 10091957

Printed by Printforce, the Netherlands

GPSR Compliance

The European Union's (EU) General Product Safety Regulation (GPSR) is a set of rules that requires consumer products to be safe and our obligations to ensure this.

If you have any concerns about our products, you can contact us on ProductSafety@springernature.com

In case Publisher is established outside the EU, the EU authorized representative is:

Springer Nature Customer Service Center GmbH
Europaplatz 3
69115 Heidelberg, Germany

Batch number: 10091957

Printed by Printforce, the Netherlands